HEALTH CARE FOR
OLDER PEOPLE

T0234509

HEALTH CARE FOR OLDER PEOPLE

Practitioner perspectives in a changing society

Steve Iliffe

*Reader in Primary Care in the Department of Primary Care and
Populations Sciences, UCL Medical School and Royal Free Hospital
School of Medicine, and general practitioner, London*

Linda Patterson

*Consultant Physician and Medical Director, Burnley Health Care
NHS Trust, Honorary University Clinical Teacher, Department of
Geriatric Medicine, University of Manchester*

Mairi M Gould

*Lecturer in Primary Care, Faculty of Health Care Sciences,
St George's Hospital Medical School and Kingston University,
London*

First published in 1998
by BMJ Books, BMA House,
Tavistock Square, London WC1H 9JR

British Library Cataloguing in Publication Data

A catalogue record for this book is available
from the British Library

ISBN 0–7279–1192–9

Contents

Authors

Dr Steve Iliffe MBBS, MRCGP is Reader in Primary Care in the Department of Primary Care and Population Sciences, University College London Medical School and Royal Free Hospital School of Medicine, and a general practitioner in North West London. His research interests include innovative primary care for older people and the psychiatry of old age.

Dr Linda Patterson MB, FRCP(Edin), FRCP(Lond) is a Consultant Physician in Medicine for the Elderly at Burnley Health Care NHS Trust, where she is also the Medical Director. She is an Honorary University Clinical Teacher, Department of Geriatric Medicine, at the University of Manchester, is a member of the Geriatrics Committee of the Royal College of Physicians of London and an elected member of the General Medical Council.

Mairi M Gould BSc is Lecturer in Primary Care Nursing at St George's Hospital Medical School and Kingston University, London. Her research interests are in promotion of physical activity in and health beliefs of older people.

Acknowledgments

We thank our colleagues in local health and social services who have provided information and have discussed their experiences of community care; and Dorothy Abel at Rossendale General Hospital and Debbie Wilson at the Royal Free Hospital Medical School for excellent secretarial support.

Introduction

Why has this book been written, who should read it, and what does it say?

We have written it because the health problems of older people are not only inherently complex but also inseparable from their social relationships and circumstances. These problems challenge clinical workers in medicine, nursing, and other professions to understand their patients in terms of the organic, social, and psychological dimensions of their lives and force us right to the limits of our professional knowledge and identity.

The services that work for older people struggle with this challenge, with varying success, and the history of health care for older people is itself a history of complex organisations striving to communicate and collaborate across boundaries that often seem impermeable.

Changes in the NHS and in social care in the past two decades have increased this complexity by introducing internal markets, screening programmes, community care, and a primary care led health service. We have written this book as a guide to best practices and policies in the most taxing discipline in modern health care—care for older people.

We hope that it will be read by clinical workers of all disciplines who work with older people, by those working in social care, by health service managers, and even by policy makers. Hopefully everyone will find something useful in it to help their work, but we do not expect anyone to agree with all of it.

The book has five themes:

(1) The aging of the population is nothing new and is by no means a disaster in the making.

(2) The older population is healthier and more active socially and economically than many health and social care workers think.

(3) The key players in the care of older people are, in order of significance:

- Older people themselves
- Those who care for them when necessary
- Social support and social care
- Community health services
- Medical care.

(4) The most underdeveloped components of clinical care for older people are multidisciplinary working and the limited knowledge and skill base in general practice—public health community trusts are underdeveloped as teams.

(5) Resources for development of care for older people are to be found within the population, both in the efforts of older people themselves and in the funding needed for high quality services.

In trying to examine these themes we have tried to remain practical, to illustrate arguments with realistic scenarios, and to offer solutions to problems. Throughout the book we have used the word "patient" without apology, preferring this term denoting "one who suffers" to its commercial rivals "client" and "customer" for reasons that the chapters make obvious.

1 Aging, illness, and disability: a rising tide?

Our society is not aging rapidly. Since 1981 there has been no increase in the proportion of the population aged 65 and over, currently standing at 16% of the total population. This age group will probably shrink to 15% of the total population by 2001 and rise to 17% by 2011.[1] The projected rate of increase among those aged 60 or more during the 1990s is 0.08% a year, about a quarter of that projected for those under 60, while the number of those aged 65 to 74 is likely to fall by half a million. The population of women aged 75 to 84 seems likely to fall by 0.6% a year in the first decade of the next century. Those aged 85 or more will constitute 12% of the older population (defined as those aged 65 or more) but only 1% of the total population.[2] The impact of this change in population structure on health and health services is difficult to predict given the almost complete absence of reliable, objective data on changing patterns of morbidity in later life in Britain.[3] Predictions suggest, however, that there may be a shift from the traditional pyramidal aging structure to one that is more cylindrical, though this depends on accurate forecasts for both mortality and fertility and the latter is less likely to be accurate.

We are living through a pause in the process of demographic aging and probably face only a modest increase in the size of the older population in the first quarter of the twenty first century, with a projected increase among those aged 60 and over from 20% to 24%.[4] Scandinavia experienced such a change in the middle of this century and contained the most stable and successful societies in Europe.

1

The aging of British society occurred during the middle decades of this century and was accommodated without hugely damaging effects on social structures or the economy. Projected increases in the proportion of older people in the population at the beginning of the next century are neither new nor unprecedented, and they will be significantly less than increases in underdeveloped countries, which will experience the greatest problems of service provision.[2] Anxieties about the aging of the British population and the effect of demography on provision of health and social services are, therefore, less to do with the absolute numbers of older people than to do with heightened expectations about the type, length, and costs of such care.

The older population is an important resource for the whole community. Changing patterns of marriage and fertility over the past 50 years have resulted in the expansion of the social networks of older people. In 1977 one third of those aged 75 or over had no children, but by the early 1990s this had fallen to nearer 16%.[5] More is demanded of older people by their children and grandchildren, and more support is offered to them, contrary to the myth that children neglect and abandon their aging parents. The result is that older people provide over a third of the so called informal care of ill and disabled people, act as a major source of child care for the increasing proportion of working mothers, and provide the backbone of voluntary support in the health service and in voluntary organisations that contribute on a broad scale to health and social care.[1] The relationship between older people and their children, friends, and neighbours is not one of simple dependency of young on old but a complex exchange relationship which shifts only gradually—and then only sometimes—towards the younger becoming the predominant givers.

The major contribution of older people to family and local economies can occur because we are not only living longer but remain healthier for longer too. Life expectancy for women is currently 79 years, and 74 for men, with projected figures of 83 for women and 78 for men by the year 2021.[1] Instead of the pandemic of disability and dementia implied in apocalyptic interpretations of demographic change, most of the gain in life expectancy seems to be occurring without disability.[6,7] A woman of 65 with 17.6 years' life expectancy will remain fit and active for nine or ten years and a man of the same age, with a life expectancy of 13.7 years, for seven or eight years. American studies of cohorts of older people during the 1980s showed that the decline in disabling conditions was most pronounced for disorders of the heart and circulation.[8] In these studies the probability that a person aged 85 or over would remain free of disabilities increased by nearly 30% during the 1980s. The impact of improving health can be seen in the recent review of the 1991 census and seven other national surveys of older people.

Getting around after 60

- Among those aged 60–79, 57% of men and 40% of women had taken part in some sporting activity in the previous month. The percentages were 21% and 12%, respectively, for those aged 80 and over age group

- About 59% of men and 64% of women aged 60–79 had no limiting long standing illness

- Half of those aged 60 and over had a conversation with a neighbour or friend every day, and 95% had such a social contact at least once a week

- Among those over 65, 80% had no difficulty with any personal care, 68% had no difficulty with any domestic task, and 69% had no difficulty with any locomotor task

- In 1987 one in six of those aged 60 and over had done some voluntary work in the previous year, as had 8% of those aged 80–84

Source: Jarvis C, Hancock R, Askham J, Tinker A. *Getting around after 60: a profile of Britain's older population.* London: HMSO, 1996.

This is not to say that Fries's theory about the compression of morbidity into the last few months of life,[9] with an active, fit existence suddenly turning into disability and fatal illness over a short period of time, has been proved true for the whole population. A considerable minority of older people have major, disabling problems that require medical, nursing, and social support if anything like normal life is to be maintained, and the prevalence of major neurological and musculoskeletal causes of disability, like stroke, the dementias, Parkinson's disease, osteoarthritis, and fractured neck of femur, is likely to rise.[10] Figure 1.1 shows the main causes of mortality among older people, and highlights the importance of cardiovascular and respiratory disease.

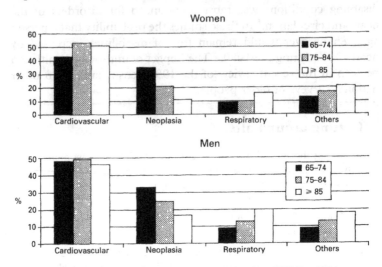

Figure 1.1   *Main causes of death by age, England and Wales, 1991*

Morbidity causing some degree of disability increases with advancing age and is more prevalent in women than in men. The major causes of disability are:

- Cardiovascular diseases, including cerebrovascular disorders
- Loss of vision and hearing
- Osteoarthritis
- Osteoporosis
- Urinary incontinence
- Depression
- Dementia.

Most of our understanding of the scope of disability comes from the General Household Survey, which uses self reported morbidity that may not reflect health status as much as people's expectations about health and the availability of services. The health status of older people may be improving, in parallel with life expectancy, and the increased use of services by older people may reflect a complex mixture of increasingly effective treatments, increasingly

4

available services, and increasing expectations of health care by professionals and the public.

Aging in consumer societies

We will return to these clinical problems and their implications for service organisation in later chapters because they do constitute a challenge to health and social care. We must, however, consider the well old too because the addition of years to life and life to years also brings with it new problems with medical implications for the relatively well and active older population. A good example of this new kind of problem is the debate about fitness to drive in later life (see box on page 6). Are older drivers "a problem", and what should be done to ensure that driving licences are issued only to those who can safely drive? The answers will have direct implications for accident and emergency services (and hence for elective surgery which may be displaced by a rise in emergency surgical admissions) and could have indirect effects on social relationships, voluntary services, and child care arrangements.

Aging as a problem

Why is the aging of the population seen as such a great problem? Theories of ageism suggest that we all have a profound prejudice against older people, perhaps because they reflect our own mortality. There is some truth in this, but for those working in health and social care there seem to be other explanations.

- Policy decisions taken with a short term perspective undermine the positive contribution of older people to society, most recently by increasing levels of poverty among pensioners.
- Services themselves are designed and organised to solve the problems of the past and find adaptation to meeting present and future needs difficult; a problem seen in the debate about age limitations on services and treatment.
- The tools available to shape planning of health services are crude and clumsy, and alternative market solutions offer no great advance for the development of services for older people.
- The professions concerned have limited ways of thinking about their work and a defensive attitude to their status, so that investigation of alternative approaches and methods is resisted.

5

Research note: fitness to drive in later life

The number of older drivers, especially those aged over 80, is increasing rapidly. The crash rate per driver among those aged over 65 is low, probably because older drivers tend to:

- Drive shorter distances
- Avoid driving at night, in heavy traffic, or in bad weather.

However, the crash rate per mile driven for older drivers is higher than that for younger adults and is lower than in only one other group, teenagers. Right of way and turning accidents are particularly common with older drivers and may reflect age related changes in vision that cause problems with:

- Merging traffic streams
- Vehicles appearing unexpectedly in their peripheral vision
- Judging own speed and that of approaching vehicles
- Reading poorly lit road signs or dim vehicle information displays

It is not clear whether these problems can be overcome or ameliorated, and the tendency of many older people is to avoid driving in situations that put them at most risk. This may not be practical for some, especially if they do have an important social role in collecting children from school, working for voluntary bodies, or even in maintaining paid employment. The increase in the pace and density of modern traffic puts older drivers at a disadvantage, but this may diminish as a generation who learnt to drive late in life gives way to one which grew up in an automotive society.

Source: Waller JA. Health status and motor vehicle crashes *N Engl J Med* 1991;**324**:54–5, Kline DW, Kline TJB, Fozard JL, *et al*. Vision, aging and driving: the problems of older drivers. *J Gerontol* 1992;**47**:27–34.

Pensions, choices, and health

A number of government policies over the past 15 years have had a negative effect on the ability of older people to remain healthy and active and to contribute to social life. Since 1980 the state national insurance pension has been linked to prices instead of to earnings, as previously, with a resultant decline in the real value

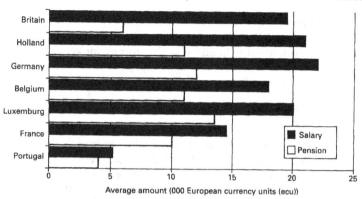

Figure 1.2 *Income replacement ratios of compulsory pension schemes 1990. Ratios are based on a pensioner with average wage in manufacturing industry and whose spouse has not worked*[12]

of the pension, which is now worth only 16% of average male earnings. As this rate is below the means tested income support level any older person receiving only the state pension is, by definition, in poverty. Two thirds of older men but only one quarter of older women have additional occupational pensions. Low income constrains personal choices in a number of ways, the most immediate being in shopping for food. A study of dietary habits and beliefs among all age groups in Cardiff showed that older people knew only slightly less about healthy eating than young people and had increased the amount of fish and fibre and decreased the amount of meat in their diet but to a lesser extent than younger people.[11] The authors speculated that older people were less likely than younger people to act on information about healthy eating because they did their shopping in ways that militated against healthy choices, possibly because lack of car ownership reduced access to large supermarkets with wide ranges of products.

Access to transport is reduced for older people, partly because car ownership is less common in older age groups, partly because of the impact of visual impairments on older drivers mentioned above, and partly because of the reduction in low cost public transport that has occurred in the past 15 years.[1]

Finally, community care policies have made it more difficult for older people to obtain local government funding for services at

7

home and state funding for residential care. This is especially true for older women living alone on low incomes, who are more reliant on outside sources of help and less able to pay for services.[12]

Case study: Mrs A

Mrs A is an 83 year old widow living on the state pension who has persistent bone pain and intermittent hypercalcaemia for which no cause can be found despite thorough investigation in the local teaching hospital. She is slowly losing weight and becoming less able to manage alone at home. After a brief inpatient episode because of a chest infection she is discharged home with a request to social services to offer her home care. Mrs A, however, has already declined the support offered—help with shopping, since her neighbour helps with housework—on the grounds of cost. The social services offered shopping at a local corner store for £3 a trip or at a distant supermarket, which Mrs A prefers on grounds of cost, at £10 a trip. Since the lower cost service implied higher food bills while the higher cost service abolished the price benefit of the supermarket, Mrs A declined both offers, and social services withdrew. During recovery for her chest infection Mrs A relied on a neighbour for shopping and housework, but illness in the family took the neighbour away from the district, and Mrs A became unable to fend for herself, ultimately falling while attempting to prepare food. She was admitted to the GP unit of the local hospital for rehabilitation and for the organisation and planning of better support; she stayed there for four weeks before returning home.

The income of older people in Britain, as a proportion of average wages in manufacturing industries, is lower than most west European nations and remains a problem both for older citizens and for service providers.

Service obsolescence

Geriatric medicine was invented to correct the neglect of older people's health that faced the NHS in the immediate period after the war. It became effective and successful as a discipline within medicine because it identified old age as a problem period needing particular responses from the NHS. As the health of older people improved, this solution itself became a problem. Old age was assumed to be a period of prolonged illness and disability for all, the older population was perceived as homogeneous in its neediness, creating crude tools for service planning for older people. For example, the underlying assumption that all older people have the same health needs was used in the formulae for resource allocation, so that a population with a large proportion of older people received proportionately more resources than one with a smaller proportion. Yet the reason for the difference in proportions of older people in different local populations was selective migration at retirement of those affluent and well enough to relocate. Small elderly populations in the inner cities may have greater health needs because they are too ill or too poor to move to seaside towns, but a resource reallocation formula based on age alone transferred funds away from the most needy to those with better health.[13]

More recent attempts to direct the development of the NHS have not moved away from the view that the older population is radically different from other age groups. The *Health of the Nation* white paper emphasises the need to reduce premature mortality, especially by reducing the rate of heart disease and stroke among those under 74, even though heart disease and stroke are the major causes of death in those aged over 75. This example reflects the neglect of the health of the older nation in NHS planning, for 10 of the 15 targets set in the *Health of the Nation* strategy are concerned with reducing premature mortality, and three of the five others with reducing the incidence of life threatening illnesses—a bias in favour of adding years to life rather than adding life to years, even though life expectancy is lengthening and the major problems of later life are those of disabling morbidity.

The statistical indicators in *Health of the Nation* often exclude older people as a target population. People aged 75 and over are excluded from all four targets for heart disease and stroke and one of the four for cancer (but mammography services are based on the 50 to 69 age group while cervical screening targets exclude those over 70). The impact of these diseases on older people is recognised but interventions are aimed at younger age groups, partly because of the limited information available about the effectiveness of intervention. This use of age cut off reflects the paucity of research on medical interventions in later life because older people tend to be excluded from clinical trials even though they have the potential to benefit directly from therapeutic and preventive strategies, sometimes benefiting proportionately more than their juniors from technological advances.[3] Work carried out in this area suggests that older people benefit more from health promotion in terms of health gain.

The evidence is mounting that no significant age difference exists in mortality or morbidity outcomes of a range of interventions, including cardiopulmonary resuscitation, coronary arteriography and bypass surgery, liver and kidney transplantation, other forms of surgery, chemotherapy, and dialysis.[14] In other words, physiological age is more important than chronological age in determining responses to treatment, rendering services organised around chronological thresholds less effective than their patients deserve, as the box below shows.

Audit point: Age and thrombolytic treatment in myocardial infarction

Older people with myocardial infarction sometimes fail to receive the treatment that younger patients get, for no apparent reason other than their age. A unit of medicine for elderly patients operating an age-related admissions policy with a threshold of 71 years began using thromboembolytic therapy in 1988 and experienced "inordinate" pressure on nursing and medical staff, especially at nights and weekends. Audit of thrombolysis among older patients with myocardial infarction two years after the introduction of the treatment showed that only five of 41 older patients received thrombolytics. A vigorous policy of staff training was introduced and a high dependency unit developed to allow trained nursing staff to monitor patients with infarcts who were receiving thrombolytic treatment. One year later a repeat audit showed that 15 out of 43 patients received thrombolytics, and six months later all eligible patients were so treated.

Source: Hajela VP, Singh SK, Patterson LJ. Thrombolytic treatment for elderly patients. *BMJ* 1992;**305**:1294.

Limits of market solutions

If planning approaches, research, and service organisation misconstrue the patterns of health and illness among older people, can market mechanisms be more sensitive and offer better tools for allocating resources for care of older people? So far the gain has been small. The division of social care along purchaser-provider lines has resulted in the introduction of means testing for services, indistinct divisions between health and social care, and reduced access to social care because of resource limitations. We shall return to this issue later in this chapter when we review the services available in the community and again in chapter 6. In medicine the introduction of economic analyses as the basis of service planning and of outcome measures that serve as a surrogate for profit—"health gain" in the jargon—have not been of great benefit to older people.[15] The hazards to older people of the use of ideas borrowed from the discipline of health economics and used by untutored professionals as tools for planning provision are shown in the box on page 12.

Given the misconceptions that abound about the health of older people and the limited amount of scientific evidence about current and likely future needs, what can those working with older people in health and social services do? Much that has been written about the impact of demographic change on health services emphasises the demands that the very old will make on community health care and hospitals so that it is easy to develop a narrow perspective on the tasks faced. This book offers a wider perspective that we hope places all the elements of care for older people in their rightful places, showing their inter-relationships, strengths, and weaknesses, and makes some proposals about future development of health and social care for older people. First, we consider the resources available to us.

The resources

The medical and social care of older people in the community in Britain depends on six agencies, which, in order of importance, are:

- Older people themselves (and their social networks)
- Social services
- Community nursing services
- General practitioners
- Hospital specialists
- Commercial residential and nursing homes.

11

Hazards of health economics

Opportunity cost

Transfer of care of older people to "informal" carers may allow money to be diverted elsewhere in medical care, reducing the opportunity costs to the health service, but only if the costs to carers are not measured or valued—including their withdrawal from the labour market.

Efficiency

Social efficiency exists when the total of outputs is maximised and it is impossible to make one person better off without making another worse off. When *aggregate* social efficiency is considered, as it may be for ease of measuring outputs, it is possible for benefit to be displaced from older people to younger, especially if older people are perceived as having had "a good innings", to be unlikely to gain from treatment, or to be an unproductive burden.

Cost effectiveness analysis (CEA)

Services are accepted in CEA if they maximise benefits for a given cost or minimise cost in the achievement of a defined benefit. One side of the equation is fixed (either cost or benefit), and this can create difficulties when a multiplicity of clinical problems coexist, especially if they include intangibles like wellbeing. For older people, whose problems may be complex and multiple, the result of this approach may be to reduce inputs to achieve a narrowly defined gain or package services within costs and define patient need in terms of such services.

We will explain in this book how these different services can collaborate for the benefit of their patients and clients and point to new developments that may overcome remaining problems in the care of older people. Firstly, each of the key agencies needs a brief introduction.

Older people themselves

Older people themselves, with their families, their neighbours, their social and cultural organisations (especially religious groups), and voluntary organisations like *Age Concern* and the *Alzheimer's Disease Society*, make a major contribution to the medical and nursing care of ill or disabled older people. Although disability increases in prevalence during the eighth decade of life, most older people are relatively well. Among those aged 75 and over, about one fifth take no medication on a regular basis, two fifths need medication regularly to control medical problems, and the remainder have multiple medical problems and use three or more medicines on a regular basis. About 80% are able to get out of their homes without assistance from others, and 95% are able to move about within their own homes independently. Their main difficulties are with bathing and with foot care, particularly cutting nails.

This large group of retired citizens has an important social and economic role in providing care for others, including child care, voluntary work in hospitals and in the community, and care for ill family members or neighbours. Their importance has been recognised—belatedly—by government, which has focused the attention of social and medical services through the Carers Act 1995, which offers special support to older people caring for others (see chapter 3).

Voluntary organisations are particularly powerful sources of information, education, and support. The *Alzheimer's Disease Society*, for example, has local branches which work to increase public awareness of Alzheimer's disease, raise funds for research, contribute to training of professionals working with Alzheimer sufferers, run support groups for people caring for those with dementia, and in some places provide assistance in the home for families.

Social services

Social services are provided by local government according to defined criteria of need, with financial contributions from the older person who uses them. These services provide:

- Help with work in the home (cleaning, shopping)
- Help with personal care (especially bathing)
- Aids to daily living (adaptations to the home like stair rails, showers in place of baths, elevated chairs that help people to rise to their feet)
- Communication systems and alarms that allow people living alone to get help easily
- Places in day centres for social and sometimes therapeutic activities

13

- Information about financial benefits that are available to those with low incomes or those who are looking after ill or disabled relatives
- Information about clubs and social activities, including physical activity programmes ("keep fit" classes)
- Access to residential care in nursing homes for short term relief of carers or for longer term care.

Local government also controls access to subsidised transport—cheap bus fares, use of taxis at subsidised costs, and dedicated bus services for disabled people. *Dial a Ride* services are provided by a large number of local authorities.

Local governments have had less and less money to spend during the past decade, with the result that these services have decreased or have been "means tested"—making older people pay for some services, like home help and personal care. The organisation of social care has also been moved on to a market basis, so that local government social service departments now buy services for older people from private agencies instead of providing services directly.

Community nursing

Community nurses work for the NHS and are employed by local organisations (usually community trusts) which are separate from local government. They include health visitors, district nurses, school nurses, and community psychiatric nurses.

District nurses take referrals from a wide variety of sources (including self or relative referral) and will assess and provide nursing care in the home at the request of general practitioners (see chapter 5) or hospital specialists (see chapter 3). This home nursing care may be complex, providing care at a level comparable with that of a hospital ward ("Hospital at Home"), or very specialised, providing care for those who are dying (Macmillan nurses and "Hospice at Home") or for those with mental health problems (community psychiatric nurses).

District nurses provide nursing care for all ages of people in the community but because of the greater needs in this age group their workload tends to focus on older people and includes daily care for those with disabilities so severe that they are unable to look after themselves unaided. District nurses also care for patients discharged from hospital after operations, and this task is increasing in importance because of rising rates of day surgery and ever shorter inpatient stays—six to seven days on average after emergency admission for major illnesses, up to 11 days after hip replacement. They are usually experienced in assessment of disability and usually have good working relationships with social services, unlike their general practitioner colleagues (see chapter 4).

General practitioners

General practitioners are doctors who provide medical care for people of all ages within a small locality. They are not employed by the NHS but they have contracts with it. People register with a general practitioner, who acts as a gatekeeper to medical specialists. General practitioners must have three years special training in a wide range of medical disciplines (including care of older people) before they can work in the community. There are 33 000 general practitioners, and on average each has 1900 registered patients, of whom on average about 130 are aged 75 and over. Most general practitioners now work in groups, with the average group size being three or four. General practitioners must provide services for their patients 24 hours a day, every day of the year, and at nights and weekends many general practitioners transfer their responsibility of care to a local cooperative of doctors.

This general medical care is provided in a clinic or in patients' homes if they cannot come to the clinic. The doctor may be assisted by nurses and psychologists and many other health and social care staff, depending on premises and funding. General practitioners are paid a fixed sum each year for each person registered with them, which is higher for those aged 65 and over than for younger people. Since 1990, every general practitioner must make an annual invitation to each patient aged 75 and over to have a health review, in the patient's home.

This review must include assessment of:

- Sensory functions, especially sight and hearing
- Mobility and the need for aids to mobility
- Mental condition
- Physical condition including continence
- Social support and environment
- Use of medication.

15

Unfortunately most general practitioners are ill equipped to do this very well, so the potential for further improving the health of older people and their quality of life is not realised. The reasons for this reluctance are complex and are reviewed in chapter 5, but include among some doctors the belief that "nothing much can be done" for disabling problems like depression, dementia, and arthritis. As a whole general practitioners have limited relationships with social services, which results in avoidable inefficiencies in providing and coordinating care. This assessment programme has not been given high priority by the NHS, and little effort is made to help general practitioners to carry it out.

Hospital specialists

Older people have access through their general practitioners to specialists in the care of the elderly in every district. Many (but not yet all) districts also have psychiatrists who specialise in old age psychiatry.

Hospital specialists in medicine for older people run outpatient clinics, wards for acutely ill older people, rehabilitation services, and in some cases also have some long stay beds for those who cannot be looked after at home. They are also able to visit ill people in their home but only at the request of the general practitioner. All district hospitals have an emergency department which may be used at any time of day by those who are acutely ill. They may also run day hospitals for assessment of ill older people and for their rehabilitation after acute illnesses and may have "outreach" services which visit older people in their homes.

The emphasis in specialist medicine for older people is to ensure rapid recovery from acute illnesses like myocardial infarction and pneumonia, to maximise recovery of function after stroke, and to increase mobility and self care among those with disabling disorders like osteoarthritis, rheumatoid arthritis, and Parkinson's disease.

Nursing homes

Commercial residential and nursing homes provide care for those older people with long term illness and disability. They have taken over the main role of providing continuing care for very frail old people from NHS hospitals, most of which have closed their wards for long term care, and from local governments, which have reduced the number of long stay homes. The costs of care in commercial nursing homes may be paid in part by the government and part by the patient or their family. This has created a problem for some older people, who have been forced to sell their houses to pay for their own care instead of passing the house to their children.

Recent successes

There have been some recent successes in the provision of care for older people in Britain.

The rapid growth of high quality specialist medical services in hospitals, during the 1970s and 1980s—This has brought effective curative medicine to older people on a wider scale than previously and is helping to overcome the belief that older people cannot benefit from advanced and high technology medicine and surgery. Medical care for older people with severe cardiovascular and respiratory disease, with severe arthritis, and for visual loss has improved significantly. Age barriers to treatment are being raised, and health promotion activities are being designed for people up to the early or mid 80s in hypertension control, smoking cessation, and physical activity.

An increase in the number of community based residential homes for frail elderly people in the same period—These homes are usually small, allowing frail and chronically ill people to stay closer to their family and neighbourhood instead of being moved to large hospitals some distance away.

The successes have helped older people with serious illness and disability enormously and cannot be underestimated. Those with less severe but still significant problems, who remain in their own homes and do not need so much specialist medical care, however, have not benefited so much.

Remaining problems

Remaining problems in the provision of medical and social services for older people are mainly problems of caring for people in the community.

17

The limited resources of local government leading to rationing of care, and the introduction of charges to patients by social services. These may prevent older people with low incomes, or with relatively less severe problems, from obtaining services. Such people may seek help from the NHS because it is free but find that it cannot meet their needs. Frail older people may be admitted to hospitals when they could be cared for at home, but lack of resources in local government prevents the deployment of the necessary social services.

The slow, uneven development of good quality care for older people in general practice—General practitioners provide services according to public demand, and older people may be less demanding than younger because:

- They have low expectations and believe that their illness or disability is "normal" for their age
- They are more respectful towards doctors and nurses than younger people and believe that there is "always someone worse off than me"
- They are less mobile and have more communication difficulties (because of deafness, for example).

This results in bias towards younger, relatively well people and against older people. A change in approach is underway in general practice, with attention to need rather than demand being emphasised, but such change is necessarily slow. The rate of change could increase if greater political priority were to be given by the NHS to the health of older people living in the community.

The different organisation of services can cause inefficiencies in organisation and poor coordination so that the quality of service deteriorates. Innovative mechanisms, or possibly even a single organisational structure, are needed to allow general practitioners, community nurse, social services, and medical specialists to work together.

Conclusions

Many attempts are being made to overcome these problems, making work with older people one of the most dynamic and exciting areas of health care. The biggest obstacle to high quality, efficient, and humane care for ill older people is probably the limited funding of local government, and this must be overcome in the next decade if the problems experienced by an aging population are to be dealt with effectively.

The issue of coordination of services is being approached from different directions, with experiments to bring together social care workers and general practitioners and to extend health promotion through collaborative work between general practitioners, specialists, and community nurses. These issues are discussed in more depth in chapters 3 and 4.

Although we are beginning to understand that the health of older people is of great importance to the whole of society, we have not yet understood how much change must take place in the attitudes of professionals, in the way in which money is spent on health and social care, and in the ways that we work together on a daily basis. The research agenda around care of older people is long and is covered again in our conclusion.

1 Arber S. Is living longer a cause for celebration? *Health Services Journal* 1996; 106:28–31.
2 Victor C. *Health and health care in later life.* Milton Keynes: Open University Press, 1991.
3 Medical Research Council. *The health of the UK's elderly population.* London: Medical Research Council, 1994.
4 Warnes AM. Elderly people in Great Britain: variable projections and characteristics. *Care of the Elderly* 1989;1:7–10.
5 Timaeus I. Family households of the elderly population; prospects for those approaching old age. *Ageing and Society* 1986;6.
6 Grimley Evans J, Goldacre MJ, Hodleinson HM, Lamb S, Savoy M. *Health and function in the third age (the Carnegie Report)* London: Nuffield Provincial Hospitals Trust, 1993.
7 Robine JM, Ritchie K. Healthy life expectancy: an evaluation of global indicator of change in population health. *BMJ* 1991;302:457–60.
8 Manton KG, Stalland E, Corder L. Changes in morbidity and chronic disability in the US elderly population: evidence form the 1982, 1984 and 1989 national long term care survey. *J Gerontol* 1995;50B:S104–204.
9 Fries JF. Aging, natural death and the compression of morbidity. *New Engl J Med* 1980;303:130–5.
10 Tallis R. Rehabilitation of the elderly in the 21st century. *J R Coll Physicians* 1992;26:413–22.
11 Vetter NJ, Lewis PA, Charny M, et al. Dietary habits and beliefs of older people. *Health Visitor* 1990;63:263–5.
12 Dall JLC. The greying of Europe. *BMJ* 1994;309:1282–5.

13 Williams ES, Scott CM. Health needs vary among elderly people. *BMJ* 1994; **309**:198.
14 Jecker NS, Schneiderman LJ. Futility and rationing. *Am J Med* 1992;**92**:191.
15 Jones IR, Higgs PFD. Health economists and health care provision for the elderly: implicit assumptions and unstated conclusions. In: Morgan K, ed. *Gerontology: responding to an ageing society.* London: Jessica Kingsley, 1992.

2 Family and other "informal" carers

Worldwide the numbers of elderly people are expected to continue growing well into the next century. The most dramatic increase is in the number of the very old—in the United Kingdom by 2001 there will be more than four million aged 75 and over and those over 85 will exceed one million. The important question is what level of disability is present in those extra years—are older people living longer and remaining fit or is an increasing proportion of later years spent in disability?

There is an association between advancing years and increasing rates of disability—more than two thirds of disabled adults (4.2 million) are aged 60 and over. Most are not severely disabled. After the age of 70 and especially over 80, however, there is a marked increase in the proportion with severe disabilities.[1]

The Office of Population Censuses and Surveys (OPCS) undertook a series of major surveys in 1989 into the extent of disability in Great Britain. They contacted 100 000 addresses, in both private households and "communal establishments"—that is, institutions of various types including hospitals—to identify those people with a disability. Once identified, the ability of disabled people to perform certain tasks was assessed to construct a scale of severity, ranging from 1 (the lowest) to 10 (the highest).

Three out of five disabled adults require help with at least one self care or household task—for example, washing all over, dressing and undressing, or vacuuming and shopping.[1] Nearly all of this help is supplied by an informal helper—usually a spouse or grown up children (including children-in-law). Both statutory and

21

The severity of disability

Severity category	Complaint giving rise to disability	Impairment
1	Deaf in one ear	Difficulty hearing someone
2	Angina/eye problem	Difficulty walking 180 m and eyesight problems
3	Spinal arthritis	Problems reaching and stretching. Cannot walk 180 m without stopping. Problems getting in and out of bed
4	Deaf in both ears	Very poor hearing. Finds it difficult to understand strangers
5	Phlebitis	Difficulty walking short distances, and climbing up and down stairs
6	Arthritis/stroke/heart condition	Limited mobility. Great difficulty reaching and stretching, and poor dexterity
7	Stroke	Falls over frequently. Difficulty walking short distances, and climbing up and down stairs. Poor dexterity. Occasionally incontinent
8	"Old age"	Behavioural problems. Severe forgetfulness. Very poor dexterity
9	Arthritis of spine/ deafness	Cannot understand people. Cannot get in and out of bed. Great difficulty hearing. Regularly incontinent. Very poor dexterity. Cannot bend over very far, and can only manage stairs with difficulty. Problems with eyesight
10	Senility	Cannot understand people. Intellectual functioning very low. Cannot manage self care. Can only manage a couple of steps. Incontinent. Behavioural problems

OPCS surveys of disability[1]

independent services help only a small proportion of the 4.5 million informal carers who look after someone age 65 and over. Two thirds are "main carers"—that is, those who are the sole carer or spend the most time caring for a dependant.[2]

Who cares ?

Women are more likely than men to be main carers and to care for a dependant outside the household. There are more women caring for elderly relatives than looking after children under five. It is the oldest carers who carry much of the heavier burden—the spouse is often the first source of care in old age and may give more than 50 hours of care a week. Most intensive caring is carried out by the family, although many friends and neighbours help out with tasks taking a few hours a week. As nearly half of those aged 75 and over live alone, much care is provided by people outside the household—usually by a daughter or daughter-in-law.[2]

The amount of care given can vary from less than a few hours a week to a full time commitment, especially when the carer lives with the dependent older person. Tasks may vary from "popping in to see if everything is all right", doing the shopping or going for the pension, and undertaking some household tasks such as laundry or cleaning through to a regular commitment of daily visits, providing regular hot meals, and provision of intimate personal care such as toileting, washing, dressing, and dealing with incontinence. Informal carers living with a very dependent adult may be providing basic nursing care, such as dressing wounds, looking after skin, administering complex medications, etc.

A large number of heavily burdened carers have other responsibilities in addition to their caring role—many are in paid employment or have dependent children. These carers, predominantly women, are therefore juggling many different demands on their time and emotions—a job, caring for their own immediate family, and caring for an elderly dependent relative.

Elderly carers, usually a spouse, often have ill health themselves—half have a long standing illness and over a third of these illnesses limit their activities. There has been an expectation in society that the spouse will be willing and able to take on caring duties. There has also been an expectation in the past that an unmarried daughter, with a job but no family, would give up work to care for her parents.

Two changes, however, have happened in recent years: there are far fewer single women than there once were and there is also more understanding that women may be pursuing a full time career in the same way as men do. Therefore the person who is expected to give up a job now may well be the married daughter or daughter-in-law who may be working part time.

Most old people do not live within 8 km of their children (visiting drops off as distances increase beyond that radius) and heavy care (over 20 hours a week) is almost exclusively provided by those who live with or very close by the person being cared for. One solution to the problems imposed by distance is for carer and old person to decide to live together. This, however, rarely seems to occur. It is more usual for children who are carers to have always lived with their parents or to have moved back in (for example, after divorce) before the need for care arose.

Little research has been done on levels of and attitudes to self care among elderly people from ethnic minorities. There is likely to be considerable variation between different ethnic subgroups and different socioeconomic classes. It is also not known how care within families is given. Patterns of family support are changing, and the assumption that the "extended family" will always look after dependent elders at home is no longer true. These families may also need support from formal agencies but may not know how to ask for it, and problems may not be recognised by professional staff. Help from neighbours may also be less available if racist attitudes are prevalent within a neighbourhood, with white neighbours less willing to help older ethnic minority elderly people.

Why care ?

Caring takes place within a relationship and may be motivated by love or duty or a mixture of both. The person who becomes the carer may be in the closest relationship—for example, a spouse—or be the most available—for example, a daughter living nearby. Often within a family one person becomes the carer and the rest of the family do not share in the task—and give little support. The carer may have had the role thrust on her or him with no discussion with other members of the family, and there may be assumptions often implicit within a family as to who is to undertake the caring role.

Most carers see caring as natural, involving varying degrees of affection (a more common claim of spouses than others), duty, and obligation. Carers may attribute their willingness to care to their marriage vows, to the wish to repay care given in childhood, to their horror of residential care, or to the lack of anyone else to do what needs to be done. The decision of relatives to care seems to be governed by kinship, sex of carer, distance, and emotional closeness.

The process whereby a relative becomes a carer can be more or less gradual or sudden and explicit. Care may spring from the day to day contacts of family life—daughters shopped for their mothers who in turn baby sat for them and gradually the balance of care shifted. If parents have always lived close to their children, care may be naturally drifted into, in contrast with children or parents moving to be nearby. A sudden event such as a stroke, however, may precipitate an older person into dependency and relatives into an unexpected caring role, which had not been foreseen.

The burdens of caring are in general voluntarily if not gladly borne and carers vary in their reactions to them. It is probably only a small minority of carers (about 10 %) who are definite that they do not wish to continue caring. Although nearly all can identify aspects of the carer's role which they find difficult or of which they would like to be relieved, they also suggest that caring has its satisfactions.[3]

Most carers, however, have not felt in a position to say no and therefore find themselves in an unexpected and unplanned situation. The complex motivations for caring, and continuing to care, result in many different emotional responses in the carers.

Burdens on carers

Carers face physical, emotional, social, and financial problems.[4,5] Carers have been reported as having a poorer level of self rated health and objectively to have higher rates of both physical and mental ill health.[3] Elderly carers may themselves have disabilities which limit their activities.[1]

The physical strain of performing heavy tasks such as lifting to transfer from bed to chair or from chair to toilet can lead to

Problems of carers

- Frustration
- Anger
- Guilt
- Tiredness
- Anxiety
- Depression
- Physical injury
- Ill health
- Loneliness
- Poverty

tiredness and injured backs and shoulders. Lack of sleep caused by broken nights getting up to attend to the needs and wants of the dependent person, who is perhaps wandering or very demanding of attention, can lead to chronic tiredness. Dealing with incontinence, particularly faecal incontinence, can be very distressing and also creates increased laundry costs. Coping with increased confusion in a dementing elderly person can be emotionally distressing, as the person once well known changes and may exhibit difficult and bizarre behaviour. The carer may grieve for the loss of the person they loved. Living with someone who is very forgetful and may constantly repeat the same phrases or questions or repeat the same movements can lead to high levels of irritation and frustration. They may frighten with aggression or by wandering. Lucid elderly people may also exhibit changes in personality, becoming withdrawn, demanding, or depressed, and this can produce a great deal of strain in carers, who feel they can never please the people they are trying to help.

Some carers feel physically isolated—they feel unable to leave their dependent relative, and their own social life may be non-existent. Loneliness can lead to anxiety and depression. Many carers have not had a holiday for many years and have lost contact with their own friends and no longer participate in former activities or hobbies.

Carers may also feel resentment towards the dependent person and then guilt or may feel guilty for not being able to look after them well enough—the feeling that whatever they do, it's not enough. They may feel guilty for finding the task difficult and therefore find it hard to admit to not coping and therefore to ask for or accept help. Children may find it difficult to be in a role of "parenting" their parents, and male carers particularly may be embarrassed by undertaking intimate personal care for a wife or mother. Daughters may find it difficult to attend to intimate bodily functions of their fathers.

Carers may feel angry at the situation they find themselves in and therefore with the dependent person themselves and angry with the system which isn't offering enough support. The anger may just be because the situation has happened at all—the carer recognises it is no one's fault but still feels angry and resentful.

The impact of caring on psychological health is related to the combination of the degree of dependency or difficulty of the elderly person, the state of health of the carers themselves, and the closeness of the past or present relationship between carer and cared·for.[3] The degree to which the carer finds the task stressful depends on their own expectations as well.[6,7] The carer's *perception* of the functioning and disability of the dependent person is an important determinant of the burden felt.

As well as a lot of complex negative emotions, however, carers may also feel a sense of satisfaction, the continuation of a loving relationship, and a strong sense of duty in the role. As well as physical and mental health problems and emotional strain, there may be financial consequences to adopting a caring role. Elderly spouses may be living on a low income and have financial worries about heating bills and food.

An additional source of income is the *Attendance Allowance*. This is a benefit for people who are mentally or physically disabled and need help with personal care or who need supervision from someone else of tasks such as dressing, personal hygiene, or getting meals. It is not means tested and does not depend on National Insurance contributions. There are two weekly rates—a lower rate if help is needed in the day or the night, a higher rate if help is needed in both the day and the night. The allowance is paid to the disabled person themselves and may be claimed if they are living alone or with another person. The disabled person may then choose to use the attendance allowance to pay the carer, although often the small amount of money just goes into the general pool of household income.

If a daughter or daughter-in-law has given up work to look after a dependent relative her income will obviously reduce. There will also be consequences for long term pensions, and many women will face an impecunious old age themselves because of not contributing to National Insurance or a private or occupational pension.

If carers are still working they may have difficulties combining their role with traditional working patterns, and employers are not always sympathetic.[8]

The *Invalid Care Allowance* is paid to people who are unable to work full time because they are caring for someone in receipt of the attendance allowance or disability living allowance (a benefit paid to people who become disabled before the age of 65 and who claim before they are 66). This benefit may be reduced if another benefit or pension is being received and must be claimed before the recipient is 65.

There are other benefits available—rent, income support, benefits for the blind, transport, and reductions for local leisure facilities.[9]

Many carers and older people are not claiming all the benefits to which they are entitled. Age Concern publish a book *Your Rights*, and more information can be obtained from the Department of Social Security helpline or local offices.

What do carers need ?

Most carers want to continue in their role, despite the demands, for a complex variety of reasons. However, they need and would like more support from formal community services.

The difficulties of carrying out personal care tasks—for example, dealing with incontinence—can cause great distress but may not be apparent to outside agencies. Disturbed nights and difficult demanding behaviour are also difficult to cope with.

Many carers want to be recognised and supported in their role by the formal agencies—for example, general practitioners, social services, etc.

They need *information* about the disabled person's illness—what is to be expected, will the condition change, what complications

---

Carers need:

- Information
- Support
- Recognition

Information is needed about:

- Diagnosis
- Prognosis
- Use of medication and its effects
- Lifting and handling
- Management of difficult problems, like incontinence and behavioural changes
- Services available
- Support groups

---

may occur, what is the likely final outcome, how long will it go on. If a particular symptom is understood to be part of the condition it may be easier to cope with—for example, "sundowning" behaviour in a dementia sufferer, when agitation increases in the late afternoon. The information needs to be in an understandable form and easily accessible. The general practitioner or hospital specialist services may be a source of information, as well as health visitors, district nurses, and social workers. The carer can also be advised to get in touch with self help groups which may supply more information and support—for example, Alzheimer's Disease Society, Parkinson's Disease Society. They may need help in accessing these organisations—for example, through the local Council for Voluntary Services.

Carers also need training and information in managing some of the tasks—for example, correct moving and handling techniques, management of continence. They need information about medication—the regimen, the reason for the particular medication, and possible side effects.

Respite care

It is the unremitting nature of caring and the amount of time devoted to looking after another person which causes the most stress, and many carers need and want a break on a regular planned basis.

Broken nights and the inability to go out and leave a disabled person even for a short time can cause chronic tiredness and frustration. Carers want and need support in arranging breaks to provide them with some respite from care. This may mean day or night sitters going into the home to enable the carer to go out or to have a night's undisturbed sleep. A place can be arranged for the elderly dependant at a day centre run by voluntary or statutory agencies or the private sector, although this may involve a cost. Longer breaks can be arranged by admitting the person to a residential, nursing home, or hospital care for one to two weeks to enable the carer to go away on holiday or just to rest at home—again there may be a financial cost. The frequency of these admissions can be increased depending on need.

Respite care, however, does have problems. There may be financial costs to pay. The dependent elderly person may not like strangers coming into the house and may make his or her views very clear to the carer. They may refuse to go to day care or may make life so difficult for the carer that it is easier for them not to send them. They may not want to go away to stay in a residential or nursing home, and carers may worry that the care will not be as personal or thorough in those settings.

Carers may therefore have difficulty in accepting respite care—they may feel anxious and guilty about "not coping" and a sense of failure. There is therefore a need for sympathetic counselling and support to enable the carer to reach the right decision for them and to have solutions which are acceptable to them. It is important that individual solutions are found which are right for the individuals concerned, so a variety of provision should be considered.

Elder abuse

Sometimes the dependent adult may be subject to ill treatment by carers—vulnerable adults can be abused, both at home by family

---

The case of Mr B

Mr B, age 79, has Parkinson's disease and his mobility and speech have been deteriorating over the past two years. He is becoming increasingly forgetful and confused, particularly at night. He lives with his wife, who helps him get up in the morning and assists him with washing and dressing. She accompanies him to the toilet to help with his clothes; he has occasional urinary incontinence. He receives the attendance allowance, and recently the district nurses have been calling weekly, although he will not let anyone other than his wife help him. He refuses to attend a local day centre and his wife has given up trying to persuade him to go. He also refuses any respite care. His wife is increasingly tired and wants a break, particularly as her nights are broken with him calling out.

---

members, neighbours, visitors, or practitioners or in institutional settings. Abuse may be described as physical, sexual, psychological, or financial.[10,11] It may be intentional or unintentional or the result of neglect. It causes harm to a person, either temporarily or over a period of time. Dependent adults are entitled to live their lives with the same civil and human rights as the rest of the population, and there are values which should underpin their care.[12] These are:

- Privacy—The right of individuals to be left alone or undisturbed and free from intrusion or public attention into their affairs
- Dignity—Recognition of the intrinsic value of people regardless of circumstances by respecting their uniqueness and their personal needs; treating with respect
- Independence—Opportunities to act and think without reference to another person, including a willingness to incur a degree of calculated risk
- Choice—Opportunity to select independently from a range of options
- Rights—The maintenance of all entitlements associated with citizenship
- Fulfilment—The realisation of personal aspirations and abilities in all aspects of daily life.

31

Any of these rights may be violated, and it may be very difficult for carers, who may be under a lot of strain, always to treat a dependent older person in a sensitive and caring way. Abuse is most likely to occur if the dependent person has communication problems, is aggressive, rejects help, or has challenging behaviour, or there are major changes in personality.

There may be a background of poor family relationships in the past, the carer may have been abused themselves by the person for whom they are now caring and roles may have been reversed—for example, a domineering parent has become dependent. Financial worries and poor housing may be causing stress, and if carers are emotionally and socially isolated, not receiving practical and emotional support from others (either family, friends, or professionals), and have little personal or private space, abuse may result. The carer may have frequently requested help from professionals but problems have not been solved and therefore frustration has built up, or the carer may be "sandwiched" between the responsibilities of caring and other responsibilities to their own children or work. Carers who are physically or mentally ill themselves or are becoming dependent on drugs or alcohol are also more likely to abuse. The dependent adult may be very demanding and careless of the feelings and needs of the carer and may be very selfish and self-centred. They may be physically or emotionally abusing the carer.

Physical abuse may be manifested in a variety of ways: signs of injury, particularly bruising in well protected areas—for example, inside of thigh, inside of upper arm—bruising which is bilateral or clustered, finger marks, burns, injuries found at different states of healing, inconsistent history of minor injuries or falls, malnutrition when not living alone, excessive medication, particularly hypnotics and tranquillisers, or underuse of prescribed medication.

Sexual abuse may be indicated by injury to the vagina or rectum, genital infection, bruising, and a change in behaviour, sometimes with overt sexual behaviour or language by the vulnerable person.

Psychological abuse is when a person is intimidated, blamed for behaviour or actions which are beyond their control, or harassed. It may be manifested by change in behaviour, passivity, insomnia or need of excessive sleep, paranoia or agitation, poor personal hygiene, and difficulties for others to gain access to the vulnerable individual or frequent missed attendance at day centres, luncheon clubs, etc.

Financial abuse may occur when the carer appropriates some or all of the dependent person's finances without their knowledge. This may leave them with insufficient means to meet their basic care needs.

A number of the indicators present should alert practitioners to consider whether abuse has occurred and should prompt an assessment of the needs of any carer who may be providing support and a review of services, if any, currently in place.

Signs of abuse

Physical

- Bruises in unusual places, such as the inside of the thigh or upper arm
- Clustered bruising
- Injuries at different stages of healing
- Unexplained burns, falls, and fractures
- Malnutrition
- Inappropriate administration of medication

Psychological

- Changes in behaviour
- Changes in sleep pattern

Sexual

- Genital infection
- Overt sexual behaviour
- Bruising or lacerations to the vagina or rectum
- Torn or stained underclothes

Financial

- Inability to pay bills
- Poor living conditions compared with assets

Abuse of vulnerable elderly people by informal carers is usually thought of as the result of a stressful situation rather than a pathological personality in the carer.[13,14]

The issue has been brought to the forefront of the professional agenda in recent years. Professionals are encouraged to monitor the situation of carers and to intervene if abuse is suspected. (Less emphasis has been placed on abuse taking place within institutional settings, by paid formal carers, where the great scandals of ill treatment and neglect were reported in the past.)

An alternative view has been expressed that the emphasis on monitoring carers to ensure that abuse has not occurred is an unwelcome intrusion and produces little benefit as intervention is seldom helpful.[15,16] Most carers, who do not abuse, are therefore placed under unnecessary surveillance. Far from abuse being a result of situational distress, characteristics in the carer are the best predictor of abuse—these may be a history of mental illness, substance misuse, and emotional or financial dependency on the part of the carer.[17]

This minority view is not widely accepted, and public policy is being implemented around the prevention of abuse by relieving carer stress. When abuse is suspected, a multidisciplinary multiagency approach is essential. Agencies need to have agreed local guidelines and adequate training for staff, who should know whom to contact if abuse is suspected.[18] A comparison of the issues around child abuse and elder abuse reveals how complex these are and how the experience gained with child abuse may not help in dealing with elder abuse.

What support can be offered ?

Health and social services professionals working with voluntary agencies can offer support to carers. Most carers are not in receipt of any support at all but want more help, both practically and emotionally.

Key professionals are the members of the primary health care team. General practitioners may have both dependent adults and carers on their list. Depression is often missed,[15] and general practitioners need to be aware of the possibility of mental health problems in carers. Carers need information which the general practitioner can give about the medical condition and prognosis of the dependent person. Community nurses are potentially an important source of information and support and can offer training in continence care and correct moving and handling procedures with advice from community physiotherapists. The provision of hoists to avoid back injury can be organised by the district nurses,

Differences between child and adult abuse (from *No Longer Afraid*[11])

Child abuse	Elder abuse
Familial context	
Relationships between victim and abuser often very new	Relationships between victim and abuser often with long history
Mutual abuse rare	Mutual abuse not uncommon
Financial motives rare	Financial motives common
Abusers less likely to have personal health problems	Abusers very likely to have personal health problems
Abusers less likely to suffer role conflict/role reversal	Abusers very likely to suffer role conflict/role reversal
Abusers less likely to have directly competing responsibilities	Abusers more likely to have directly competing responsibilities
Family forsees positive future: with increasing age child will become independent	Family forsees negative future: with increasing age elder will become more dependent
Societal context	
Positive stereotype of children (cute, promising)	Negative stereotype of elders (awkward, burdensome)
Status high—children are our future	Status low—elders are our past
Nuclear family well established	No sociological precedent for familial care of very elderly people by elderly children
Public has a concept of parenting that includes "good" and "bad" parents	Poor public knowledge of what constitutes good care of elderly people
Public/political demands for high practice standards in Social Service Departments	Problems not seen as priority by public or politicians for any attention at all, let alone high practice standards
Professional/legal context	
Strong body of UK research	Little UK research
Definitions largely agreed nationally	No nationally agreed definition

---

Differences between child and adult abuse (from *No Longer Afraid*[11]) *continued*

Strong legal framework	Ineffective, fragmented legal framework
Victims powerless in face of legal process	Victims can (and often do) refuse help
Structured provision of primary health care	No structured primary health care
Victims are subject to compulsory school attendance	Victims can be hidden from all but the abuser
High incidence of qualified staff in child care services	Preponderance of unqualified staff in elderly services
Good knowledge of issue at senior management level	Poor knowledge of issue at senior management level

---

Practice points

General practitioners need to . . .

- Recognise the role of carers
- Be aware of stress in carers
- Be vigilant about carers' problems, especially depression
- Give appropriate information about the disabled person's condition
- Give information about management of clinical problems
- Work with other members of the primary health care team
- Refer to other agencies
- Give information about support groups and other organisations
- Consider starting a carers' support group in the practice

---

as well as advice about the proper beds, correct mattresses, and commodes. These may be supplied through the community loans store.

Community occupational therapists can offer advice on adaptations to living accommodation and arrange for provision of aids such as wheelchairs, grab rails, etc. There may be difficulty in arranging structural alterations and delivery of certain aids, however, if cash limited budgets of local authorities and housing departments have been exceeded.

Coordination is essential, and it is preferable if one member of the primary health care team can be the key worker. This may be the district nurse, the general practitioner, the health visitor, or the social worker.

Good communication and fostering of multidisciplinary working within the team is required. Regular primary health care team meetings when complex cases are discussed can help this. The practice may do an audit of carers and decide to set up a carers' support group and display relevant information for carers in prominent places in the surgery.

The local authority social services department has the lead role in coordinating care for a dependent older person. Carers may also have an assessment under the new legislation. Practical support with household tasks can be offered, although if a carer is actually living in the same house as the dependent adult, there is often an assumption that they will carry out all such tasks, and statutory support is often not offered.

The older person might need help in getting out of bed in the mornings or back to bed at night and either district nurses or care workers employed by social services can be put in to help. Local variations may exist about which tasks are taken up by health professionals and which by social services staff, and this can be confusing to the recipient of services.

The important thing is that the situation is kept under regular review as carers' needs change. Carers need to be regarded as partners by professionals also caring for the dependent adult, and their needs and wants taken into account.

Information and support can be given by the voluntary sector, either arranged in partnership with social services or directly by the carer. Carers may also individually arrange for help to be provided by the private sector if they have sufficient financial resources. The organisation of respite care, either for a day or for longer periods, is an important task for professionals.

Professionals need to be trained in the needs of carers and to be aware of the emotional and physical problems which may result from a caring role. They need to understand the roles of other professionals so the carer can be diverted to the appropriate person and how to access the necessary information—for example, on

Useful organisations

Age Concern England, 1268 London Road, London SW16 4ER

Carers National Association, 20/25 Glasshouse Yard, London EC1A 4JS

Help the Aged, St. James Walk, London EC1 0BE

Elder Abuse Response Line—0181 679 7074 (run by Action on Elder Abuse)

Department of Social Security Leaflets Unit, PO Box 21, Stanmore, Middlesex HA7 1AY

Department of Social Security Benefits Help Line—0800 666 555

Disability Benefits Helpline—0800 882 200

Local Citizens Advice Bureau

Local Council for Voluntary Services

Alzheimer's Disease Society, Gordon House, 10 Greencoat Place, London SW1P 1PH

Stroke Association, CHSA House, Whitecross Street, London EC1Y 8JJ

Parkinson's Disease Society, 22 Upper Woburn Place, London WC1H 0RA

Arthritis Care, 18 Stephenson's Way, London NW1 2HD

Royal National Institute for the Blind (RNIB), 224 Great Portland Street, London, W1N 6AA

Royal National Institute for Deaf People (RNID), 19–23 Featherstone Street, London EC1Y 8GL

Royal Association for Disability and Rehabilitation (RADAR), 12 City Forum, 250 City Road, London EC1V 8AF

Disabled Information and Advice Line (DIAL UK), Park Lodge, Saint Catherine's Hospital, Tick Hill Road, Doncaster DN4 8QN

benefits. They also need training to recognise the signs of elder abuse. This training can be offered on special courses, by specialist health or social service professionals, or as part of the in house training for social services and health service staff, often run between the agencies. General practitioners and community trust staff need to ensure that members of the primary health care team, including themselves, avail themselves of any local training which is offered. Much information can also be gained from the many publications available about the needs of carers.[5]

Some carers find carers' support groups helpful; these may be arranged by interested individuals or supported by health, social service, or voluntary sector workers. Many carers find it hard to get away to attend meetings, however, and the uptake on these groups may not be as high as anticipated.

The Carers Act

New legislation to support carers was enacted in 1995 in The Carers' (Recognition and Services) Act. The white paper *Caring for People* had as its second key objective "to ensure that service providers make practical support for carers a high priority" and that "assessment of care needs should always take account of the needs of caring family, friends and neighbours".

The act is concerned with carers who are either providing or intending to provide a substantial amount of care on a regular basis—the carer is entitled, on request, to an assessment when the local authority is also carrying out an assessment of the person cared for in respect of community care services. As many local authorities already offer carers an assessment and take into account their views when assessing the needs of the person cared for, the legislation in effect enshrines good practice into statute. It is for local authorities to make a judgment as to what "*substantial*" and "*regular*" mean as these definitions are not laid down in the legislation. The local authorities will look at what type of tasks the carer does or will undertake, how much time is or will be spent, how much supervision does the cared for person require to manage their life, and is this or will it be a continuing commitment for the carer? The assessment must be formal and needs to be documented and mutually understood. If a user refuses an assessment, then the carer does not have a right to request an assessment as the fact that the user is being assessed is the trigger for the carer's assessment.

The assessment of carers' needs may produce a conflict with the wants and needs of the person being cared for. The older person may want to continue living at home and to avoid institutional care; the carer may be finding the burden of caring for the person intolerable, despite being given help. Whose interests are paramount?

39

The caring role will come to an end by the death of the dependent person or by the move to institutional care. The decision to stop caring is a difficult one and the carer will need ongoing support. Carers are more likely to accept the idea of residential care if:

- The carer and elderly person were not married to each other
- The carer and elderly person did not live together
- They did live together but had done so for less than 10 years
- The old person presented a variety of difficult problems and the carer did not feel emotionally close to the elderly person (a situation strongly related to whether they had felt cared for themselves in the past).[3]

There is evidence that where no more than ordinary services were being provided, the mental health of those caring for confused and very dependent old people improves, on average, if their dependant goes into a residential home or hospital.[19]

Relatives become increasingly willing to consider residential care for an old person as the latter's disability or confusion increases. This is particularly true for older people with mental impairment.

There may, however, be feelings of guilt if there is a final move into residential, nursing home, or hospital care as many older people will have stated a preference for staying at home and the carer may feel they have failed if that is no longer possible. There is evidence that carers still feel emotionally stressed, even if the practical day to day caring tasks are no longer required. Time may still be spent in daily visiting, often negotiating public transport, which may cause physical stress to older relatives.

Bereavement counselling may be needed after the death of the dependent person, and if a carer has lost all social contact or given up a job to take on the caring role there will be a big gap to be filled. Rebuilding a social life after years of isolation can be difficult, and support will be needed. Financial problems may also occur if the caring role stops. The allowances paid for caring will cease, and if a carer has given up work they will need to apply for other benefits. There may also be problems if a daughter, son, or other relative is living with the dependent person in a house owned by the older person—the assets of the house can be used to support the costs of institutional care and theoretically the son or daughter could become homeless if the house is sold (spouses are allowed

The case of Mrs C

Ten years ago Mrs C, now aged 82, suffered a severe stroke, leaving her paralysed on the left side and unable to walk or transfer from bed to chair or toilet. She regained her speech and is mentally alert. Her unmarried daughter gave up a good job to move in with her mother to look after her. Regular respite periods are given in hospital, district nurses call once a week, and she attends day care for respite twice a week.

Over the years Mrs C has become more demanding of her daughter's attention and does not like to be left. Her weight has increased and moving her is difficult, but Mrs C does not like using a hoist. Her daughter has injured her back and shoulder in lifting her.

The daughter is finding the situation increasingly stressful, although she does not want her mother to go into permanent institutional care. She is fearful of the future, faces financial insecurity, and has given up all her hobbies and friends. The hospital and day care centre staff give her a lot of personal support and opportunities to talk. She has recently been referred for counselling to a social worker to help her to consider her options for the future.

to continue to live in the marital home, although the assets may be released later).

Sometimes the carer may die before the older person being cared for. The normal grief reaction may then be exacerbated by feelings of guilt—"why didn't I go first"—and worries about the practicalities of the future. Bereavement counselling and support for the older person and the rest of the family needs to be sensitively handled and complex emotions understood to help the older person come to terms with what has happened and to make appropriate plans for the future.

The future

The legislation of the 1990 act and 1995 act seems to recognise the importance of informal caring. The reliance on a huge contribution by unpaid carers does relieve the overall costs to the welfare system, but the continued availability of family care for disabled people cannot be taken for granted. Rising rates of divorce make care more problematic—will the ex-daughter in law care for her ex-husband's parents?

Demographic changes mean there are fewer unmarried daughters, who were regarded as the "traditional carers", although their actual numbers have always been quite small. More married women in the workplace may reduce their availability to care, although half work part time. More elderly people are divorcing as well: projections predict a fivefold increase in divorce in those over 65.

Attitudes to care are also slowly changing. Studies among the public have found a low level of support for informal care; most people wanted community based professional care and were unwilling to place the major burden of care on informal carers.[20][21] The sense of obligation and responsibility may be shifting, and in the future people may be less willing to take on the role of informal carer. Older people's attitudes are also changing; they do not want dependence on children or to be a burden, although they also do not want to move into institutional care.

The future acceptance by society of the reliance on informal care is therefore uncertain, although there is also a reluctance to increase public expenditure on welfare provision and statutory services.

1 Martin J, Meltzer H, Elliot D. *The prevalence of disability among adults*. London: HMSO, 1989. (OPCS surveys of disability in Great Britain: report 1.)
2 Green H. *General household survey 1985: informal carers*. London: HMSO, 1988.
3 Levin E, Sinclair IAC, Gorbach P. *Families, services and confusion in old age*. Aldershot: Gower, 1989.
4 Jones DA, Peters TJ. Caring for elderly dependants: effects on the carers' quality of life. *Age Ageing* 1992;21:421-8.
5 Travers AF. Carers. *BMJ* 1996;313:482-6.
6 Jones DA. *A survey of carers of elderly dependants living in the community*. Cardiff: University of Wales, 1986.
7 Sinclair I, Parker R, Leat D, *et al. A review of research on welfare provision for elderly people*. London: HMSO, 1990.
8 Department of Health. *Employees and carers*. London: DOH, 1993.
9 Teale C. Money problems and financial help. *BMJ* 1996;313:288-90.
10 Bradley M. Elder abuse. *BMJ* 1996;313:548-50.
11 Department of Health, Social Services Inspectorate. *No longer afraid. The safeguard of older people in domestic settings*. London: HMSO, 1993.
12 Department of Health. *Homes are for living in*. London: DOH, 1989.

13 Age Concern, British Geriatrics Society, Carers National Association, Help the Aged, Police Federation. *Abuse of elderly people. Guidelines for action.* London: Age Concern England, 1990.
14 Social Services Inspectorate. *Confronting elder abuse.* London: HMSO, 1992.
15 Macdonald AJD. Do general practitioners "miss" depression in elderly patients ? *BMJ* 1986;**292**:1365–7.
16 Biggs S. Elder abuse and the policing of community care. *Generations Review* 1996;**6**:2–4.
17 Pilemer K, Wolf R. *Elder abuse: conflict in the family.* Massachusetts: Auburn House, 1986.
18 Owen A, Owen S. Tackling abuse of older people. *Health Visitor* 1995;**68**:493–5.
19 Challis D, Chessum R, Chesterman J, *et al.* Community care for the frail elderly: an urban experiment. *British Journal of Social Work* 1988;**18** suppl:13–42.
20 Carers National Association. *Who cares? Perceptions of caring and carers.* London: Carers National Association, 1996.
21 Joseph Rowntree Foundation. *Meeting the cost of continuing care: public views and perceptions.* 1996. Social Care Research 84.

Further reading

Working with Carers—a resource pack for general practitioners (1994), from North Yorkshire Health Authority, 3rd Floor, Ryedale House, 60 Piccadilly, York YO1 1PG

Age Concern fact sheets and *Caring in a Crisis*, from Age Concern

The Carer's Companion, by Richard Carney, (1994) from Winslow Press, Telford Road, Bicester OX6 OTS

Caring for Someone at Home, by Gail Elkington and Jill Harrison, published by Hodder and Stoughton (1996). Available from Carer's National Association

Caring at Home, by Nancy Kohner, published by National Extension College (1992)

The 36-hour Day, by N L Mace, PV Robins, BA Casterton, C Clarke, and E McEwan, published by Hodder and Stoughton (1996)

3 Community social services

Community social services have undergone a massive reorganisation recently, after the government white paper *Caring for People* in 1989 and the introduction of legislation incorporating the proposals in the NHS and Community Care Act 1990. The changes were implemented in 1993. Few clinical workers seem to understand them, and this chapter aims to summarise and clarify recent developments. There had been concern for some time about the ever increasing costs to central government of residential care for elderly people and the increasing fragmentation of services.

Recent changes

The 1980s witnessed a dramatic growth in the number of places for elderly people in private residential establishments and in private nursing homes—the rate of growth in the number of homes was even more pronounced. This massive growth can mainly be attributed to changes in the social security system which took place in 1980 and 1983. The whole of the supplementary benefits scheme was drastically revised in November 1980; there were some apparently minor alterations concerning the payment of board and lodging allowances to residents in private and voluntary sector residential homes. Such allowances had been available to those without adequate means since 1948, but the amount had been set by reference to the prevailing local charges, higher rates were discretionary. Thus there was no certainty that the supplementary benefits system would pay enough to enable an elderly person to meet the fees in a private sector home, and any assessment of their case could be made only after they had been admitted.

The crucial changes made in 1980 were to interpret the "reasonable" board and lodgings allowance as that which was equivalent to prevailing charges in private and voluntary residential sectors, the discretionary element became an automatic payment to needy elderly people in residential homes, and there was an assurance that higher fees would be met if there was a shortfall if special factors made it unreasonable for the resident to move to a cheaper establishment. Local officers, confronted by having to decide if it was reasonable to require an elderly person to move elsewhere, rarely insisted that they should. Therefore a new market of poorer elderly people was created, who would be eligible for board and lodgings payments sufficient to meet the cost of care in private residential and nursing homes—proprietors were guaranteed a source of reliable income and virtually no control existed over admissions or fees.

There was also a reduction at this time in the growth of local authority residential accommodation. The number of hospital beds occupied by the chronic sick or "long stay" geriatric and psychogeriatric patients also began to reduce as the turnover of patients through these services increased with a more aggressive approach to diagnosis, treatment, and rehabilitation. The stage was therefore set for a massive increase in private sector provision of both nursing and residential care, which was given a further boost by changes to the social security regulations in 1983, which set "reasonable" weekly charges in residential care homes for the elderly and private nursing homes. These levels were still subject to local interpretation, and there was an upward pressure on fees payable.

Central government was therefore liable for a huge increase in expenditure in paying for elderly people in residential and nursing homes who were eligible for social security payments—these constitute about a half of the residents in the private sector.

It was clear that the free run of market forces could not be allowed to prevail without creating additional pressure on the public sector. The government therefore had to seek control over central expenditure on the private residential and nursing homes sector. The Firth Committee was set up, where the principal task was to make recommendations for a coherent system of financial support for elderly people in residential care; it reported in 1987.[1] In 1986 the Audit Commission on Community Care had also reported and reached similar conclusions.[2] These were that the financial arrangements for supporting residential care were working in a way directly opposing previously stated community care policies. The number of elderly people in residential care had grown dramatically, and there were perverse incentives to place older people in institutional care rather than meet the budget demands in local authorities of providing domiciliary or day care. There were also incentives for the health service to reduce expenditure on long stay beds and place people in the private sector when they could access central government funding through social security payments.

Aims of community care

- To keep older people at home
- To promote independence
- To strengthen primary health and community services
- To strengthen voluntary and neighbourhood support

The often stated policy aims of community care to keep older people living independently at home for as long as possible and to strengthen primary and community care services with voluntary and neighbourhood support were being subverted by the financial arrangements for institutional care. Relatives, hospitals, and local authorities all had a financial interest, if no other, in the admission of elderly people to private or voluntary homes. Both the Audit Commission and the Firth report proposed that local authorities should be made responsible for funding services for elderly people and that services should be coordinated to clarify areas of responsibility between agencies.

In 1986 the government invited Sir Roy Griffiths, the chairman of Sainsbury's, to look into arrangements for community care, and he reported in 1988.[3] He recommended that local social services departments should be the lead authority for assessing community care needs in the locality and for arranging the purchase of non-health care services (not necessarily to provide these themselves). To enable this to happen, local social service authorities should meet the cost of care for people unable to afford it themselves, and the money should be transferred from central government to local government to enable this to happen. There was a requirement for good collaborative interagency working, and Griffiths recommended there should be a minister for community care.

To the surprise of many, considering the government's antipathy to the role of local authorities, most of the Griffiths proposals were incorporated into the white paper *Caring for People*, published in 1989,[4] and legislation was enacted in 1990 (The National Health Service and Community Care Act 1990). The exception was that the government did not create a minister for community care.

Caring for people

Community care services should:

- Be flexible and respond sensitively to the needs of individuals and carers
- Allow a range of options for consumers
- Intervene no more than is necessary to foster independence
- Concentrate on those with greatest need

The focus of the white paper was to clarify roles and responsibilities, bringing together the relevant sources of finance, delegating decision making to the local levels, improving accountability, and providing the right incentives.

The six key objectives for service delivery were:

- To promote the development of domiciliary day and respite services to enable people to live in their own homes whenever feasible and sensible
- To ensure that service providers make practical support for carers a high priority
- To make proper assessment of need and good case management the cornerstone of high quality care

47

- To promote the development of a flourishing independent sector alongside good quality public services
- To clarify the responsibilities of agencies and so make it easier to hold them to account for their performance
- To secure better value for taxpayers' money by introducing a new funding structure for social care.

It was recognised that existing funding structures had worked against the development of domiciliary services, and the emphasis was to be on targeting home based services on those people whose need for them was greatest. Assessment of care should always take into account the needs of caring family, friends, and neighbours. Packages of care should be designed in line with individual needs and preferences. The social services authorities were to be "enablers" and to make maximum possible use of private and voluntary providers with the stated aim of increasing the range of options and widen consumer choice. The confusion of responsibilities of different agencies had contributed to poor overall performance. The aim was that social security payments should not provide any incentive in favour of residential and nursing home care.

Caring for people

Social services authorities were to be "enablers" and to make maximum possible use of private and voluntary providers with the stated aim of increasing the range of options and widen consumer choice

---

The major changes in the white paper were as follows:

- Local authorities were to be responsible, in collaboration with other agencies, for assessing individual need, designing care arrangements, and securing their delivery within available resources.
- Local authorities should be responsible for producing clear plans for community care services, consistent with plans of health authorities.
- Local authorities have to make maximum use of the independent sector.

- A new funding structure for those seeking public support for residential and nursing home care would be introduced, with local authorities taking responsibility for the financial support; money would be transferred from the social security budget centrally to local authorities.
- The difference in payments of income support and housing benefit between people living in their own homes or in independent residential or nursing homes would be abolished (but not for those in local authority residential homes).
- Local authorities would be required to set up arms length inspection and registration units.
- A new specific grant should be made to promote the development of social care for seriously mentally ill people.

There was no ring fencing of community care money, and local authorities had to manage the funds within their overall budget. It could therefore be argued that the change in the funding arrangements was a way of capping an element of public spending rather than meeting community care needs.

Caring for people

Packages of care were to be designed to meet the needs of individuals—people were no longer expected to fit into services already provided but services should be responsive to individual needs

---

The key operational change was to design packages of care to meet the needs of individuals—people were no longer expected to fit into services already provided but services should be responsive to individual needs. Local authority social services departments have therefore introduced arrangements for assessment of needs to deliver social care to individual people.

Needs' assessment is an integrated assessment system that offers a graded response according to the type and level of need and forms part of the care management approach. Previously, service linked procedures had predetermined assessment outcomes—for example, assessment for domiciliary, day, or residential care. However, there is often a disparity between assessed needs and currently available services. A further organisational change was therefore introduced to separate the responsibility for assessing need from that of delivering or managing services. Local authorities have to place 70% of their contracts with providers in the independent sector. The separation of the purchaser from the provider involved changes in social service organisation.

Care management

Social services departments in local authorities had to devise systems of care management. Care management is the process of tailoring services to individual needs. (The original phrase was case management but this is thought to be demeaning to the individual and misleading in that it is the care and not the person that is being managed.)

Caring for people

Six key objectives:

- To promote domiciliary day and respite care
- To make practical support to carers a priority
- To use care management and assessment of need
- To promote the independent sector
- To clarify interagency responsibilities
- To change the funding structure for social care

The process can be described in seven stages: publishing information; determining the level of assessment; assessing need; planning of care; implementation; monitoring; and review.[5] All or most of the tasks may be undertaken by a single practitioner, known as a care manager, employed by social services or they may be performed by different practitioners.

1 Publishing information

Care management is about empowering users and carers to enable them to make decisions about the services they receive and to be more in control of the process through which they gain access to services. Carers and users therefore need information. Local authorities are required to publish community care plans and information about complaints procedures. They must also publish

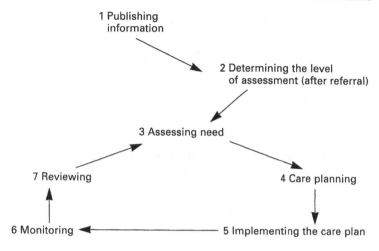

Fig 3.1

information about the types of services, criteria for providing services, and details of referral assessment and review procedures, which is accessible and easily understood. Particular care must be taken to make information accessible to users who have a language other than English, communication difficulties, or sensory impairment.

2 Determining the level of assessment

An initial identification of need is made and the appropriate level of assessment is carried out for that need. An inquiry will present to the local authority in a variety of ways—either from a user, a carer, or through other agencies. Initial information will be gathered, perhaps with a standardised referral form, to establish as quickly and sensitively as possible the urgency, level, and complexity of needs. Simple direct services such as allocation of a bus pass can be dealt with at this stage. This process should be welcoming, positive, proactive, and informed.   In many cases the presenting request can be taken at face value, but all those involved in collecting or analysing the initial information must be alert to indications of more significant difficulties. Such triggers which

51

might uncover other needs warranting more comprehensive assessment or referral to another agency may include a recent bereavement, a recent relocation to other accommodation, living alone, loss of memory, incontinence or falling, history of mental health problems, history of drug or alcohol abuse, stressed carers, or the person living on income support.

Example of information on standardised assessment form

Personal details
Referring agency/person
Is person aware of referral?
Next of kin
Main carer
Preferred communication (language/sign)
Relevant physical/mental health/mobility problems
Home details
Other agencies involved
General practitioner
Has the person had information about advocacy?
Reason for referral
Agreement to pass on information to other agencies
Action taken
Administrative coding

Assessment can then be tailored to meet the presenting need. Each authority has its own levels of assessment according to its policies, priorities, and available staff but will range from simple assessment, involving a single agency; limited assessment, meeting low risk defined needs; multiple assessment, meeting a range of needs; or assessment of complex cases with a comprehensive assessment involving several agencies and specialist professional staff. It should be clear what sort of cases will be referred for which sort of assessment.

Generally, most referral assessments fall into four categories:

● Those for whom community living is no longer a possibility or who are at risk—for example, people with intensive personal care needs

- Those who are reliant on others for survival, requiring help with, for example, feeding and toileting
- Those who rely on others for support requiring help with, for example, cleaning and shopping
- Those whose functioning or morale is reduced—for example, as a consequence of a depressive illness.

3 Assessing need

The major change here was to treat the assessment of need as a separate exercise from consideration of the service response, requiring a significant change in attitude of most practitioners.

The assessment process should be as simple, speedy, and informal as possible and be fully participative for users and carers. Users and carers should be given the opportunity to use independent advocacy if they cannot represent their own interests. It should be clear who is to do the assessment—for example, a qualified social worker—and when referrals should be made to other agencies for assessment of needs—for example, health. Comprehensive assessments that use a lot of resources are reserved for a minority of users who have complex or several needs. Sometimes users or carers themselves may present with a solution already in mind—for example, going into residential care. It is essential that a full assessment of needs is made to see if that is the best option or whether the needs can be met in another way. Such a case would probably need a complex assessment, requiring professionals from other agencies not just social services.

The practitioner should aim to reach a degree of consensus with the user as to what the real needs are; there may occasionally be differences, which need to be acknowledged and recorded. There may be disagreement between users and carers, and it may be appropriate to offer carers the opportunity of a separate assessment of their needs.

The use of the phrase "needs assessment" presumes there is an understanding of the word need. Need is a relative concept—in the terms of the community care legislation it is defined as the requirement of individuals to enable them to achieve, monitor, or restore an acceptable level of social independence or quality of life as defined by the particular care agency or authority. It is thus defined in terms of what the professionals see as the need, taking into account the views of users. Obviously changes in national legislation, local policy, availability of resources and patterns of local demand will vary the definition of need, which is thus dynamic. Need, however, is also a personal concept; no two people will perceive or define their needs in exactly the same way. The challenge to practitioners in care management is to recognise that whilst working within the constraints of local policy and resources.

Needs can be subdivided into six broad categories:

- Personal/social care
- Health care
- Accommodation
- Finance
- Education/employment/leisure
- Transport/access

Taking into account the applicant's own perception of needs, the assessment will cover these broad areas in varying degrees of detail. Each person will have his or her own attitudes and abilities and lifestyle, and these should be respected. Racial and cultural diversity should also be acknowledged. Basic activities of daily living such as eating, bathing, dressing and mobility and tasks such as shopping, using the telephone, dealing with money, and cooking should be assessed. A person's maximum ability may not be carried through into performance if there are problems with insight or motivation and this will influence the person's capacity to achieve, maintain or restore self care.

The request for social care may arise from problems in physical or mental health. Problems of memory loss may be easily overlooked as these are often accompanied by other problems such as loss of weight and may be seen by the family not the user. There may also be problems with the correct use of medication by a confused person. The appropriate involvement of health staff through consultation with the general practitioner—for example, involvement of community psychiatric nurse, approved social worker or mental health officer, or psychiatric consultant—is then essential.

Knowledge of the individual person's history, with relevant life events and coping strategies, can also form part of the assessment if volunteered by the user. Needs of carers should be assessed and may form the basis of a separate assessment if there are tensions between users' and carers' needs. Needs have to be understood in their social context, and an assessment may take into account the wider social network. Many people will already be receiving services, and the appropriateness and acceptability of these will be reviewed. Housing is important in terms of cost, adequacy, suitability, and location. If there are needs identified, housing authorities and other providers should be involved in seeking solutions to problems.

It is important to ensure that potential users are in receipt of all their benefit entitlement, and advice on handling money, if necessary, as a standard part of an assessment. Consideration of financial means will be necessary to determine the level of contribution to any service which is provided; this has to be handled tactfully, many people resent having their finances assessed. Transport needs, for example to get to the shops, should also be assessed, but are often overlooked.

Shared goals and goal setting—The needs of an individual as judged by themselves may be different from the needs as judged by their family or by a practitioner. An evaluation of risk is therefore essential. There may be environmental hazards—for example, elderly confused people with gas fires or gas cookers, poor health leading to falls or confusion, and behavioural problems such as wandering or forgetfulness or not eating adequately. These risks may be apparent to others but not to the person concerned because of loss of insight. Subject to the user's capacity to take informed decisions, however, the assessment should respect the user's entitlement to self determination and independence and be guided by self evaluation of risk. Others, for example families, may wish to be more protective of the users. The definitions of acceptable risk are difficult, but attempts should be made to be explicit and to clarify differences between agencies and professionals.

Assessment of risk

Confusion
Falls
Wandering
Poor eating habits
Environmental hazards

---

4   Care planning

This is to identify the most appropriate ways of achieving the objectives identified by the assessment of need and incorporating them into an individual care plan. Care plans will vary according to the complexity of identified needs, but the needs must be matched to the available resources. Simple needs may be met by a single service and therefore care planning can be swiftly accomplished. If continuing services are needed, all users should be in receipt of a care plan. Very complex care plans may be needed to meet complex needs, involving coordination from a number of different agencies.

The assessment should have made priorities of the users' needs and the care plan should take into account the pattern of the users' normal living, their preferences, and an assessment of acceptable risk. The aim, for most users, is to promote their independence; informal networks of care can be built into the care plan and a review of existing services undertaken. Care planning should not be seen as matching needs with services "off the shelf", but rather as an opportunity to rethink service provision for a particular individual. It is essential that there is one key worker acting as the care manager—this is usually a professional from social services, although this need not necessarily be the case. The care manager may or may not hold the budget but nevertheless should arrange for an accurate costing of the care plan, with the user being informed of any charge to themselves. Local authorities cannot charge for the process of care management and assessment but have the discretion to levy charges on services, subject to the users' ability to pay. Users may also be required to "top up" payments for certain services if they are more expensive than the financial entitlement from the local authority. If several different agencies are involved the different parts of the care plan must be integrated into a whole—this may necessitate having a meeting of all the parties.

Care plan

Should contain the following :

- The overall objectives
- The specific objectives for
  - Users
  - Carers
  - Service providers
- The criteria for measuring the achievement of these objectives
- The services to be provided by which person/agency
- The cost to the user and the contributing agencies
- The other options considered
- Any point of difference between the user, carer, care planning practitioner, or other agency
- Any unmet needs identified
- The named person responsible for implementing, monitoring, and reviewing the care plan
- The date of the first planned review

The user needs to know the name of the practitioner responsible for the implementation, monitoring, and review of the care plan. Unmet needs should also be documented and prioritised. The whole care plan should be set out in concise written form and be accessible to the user, who should have a copy. The care plan can also be shared with other agencies, who must be bound by the principles of confidentiality.

5 Implementing the care plan to secure the necessary resources or services

The aim should be to achieve the stated objectives of the care plan with the minimum intervention necessary. It should therefore seek to minimise the number of service providers involved. In some care management projects this has been achieved by introducing generic care workers who perform a range of tasks which have traditionally been divided between home care and auxiliary nursing staff.

One person, preferably the person responsible for devising the care plan, should be responsible for the implementation. There may be a conflict of interest if the care manager is also managing or delivering some of the services, although this will be inevitable with some staffing structures within local authorities.

6 Monitoring to support and control the delivery of the care plan on a continuing basis

The implementation of the care plan must be monitored to ensure that what has been planned actually happens and is still meeting the user's needs. Users and carers are the best people to comment on the services they are receiving and the care manager should support that input. The care manager will need to ensure that coordination between agencies and services is adequate, that the quality of care is acceptable, and that the cost is contained within the planned budget and to support users and carers by counselling, charting progress, and resolving conflicts.

In some care management schemes very simple accounting schemes have been developed to enable care managers with little financial training to manage budgets effectively.

7 Reviewing the care plan

Changing needs have to be identified and services adapted accordingly, taking into account the views of users and carers and the cost effectiveness of the service. If the aim of a care plan is to promote independence, success may be measured by the capacity of the individual to cope without services. Also, needs can be redefined by a change in policy of the service and targeting those in greater need may mean the reduction or withdrawal of services to some elderly people receiving them. Reasons for changing services, including withdrawal, should be fully explained to users.

It can be seen that effective care management is a complex process involving an in depth knowledge of needs assessment by a range of professionally qualified staff who have knowledge of the range of potential services and community resources available. Good interagency cooperation and skills in multidisciplinary working are essential and are perhaps the greatest challenge facing both hospital and community staff. Defined responsibilities for each agency and particular professional roles in any individual case need to be clearly understood.

Care management had been implemented for several years before *Caring for People* in some experimental community care projects, for example in Kent, where a named individual was given responsibility for constructing a "package" of services suitable to meet the needs of particular elderly people.[6] There was also a scheme to pay volunteers to provide care. Provision of flexible appropriate combinations of care did gradually reduce the likelihood of old people on the margins of residential care being admitted to a local authority home.

The Kent Community Care Project was replicated in Gateshead with similar results.[7] Care management was applied to a group of frail elderly people, one third of whom may have been expected to die in a year, and one third to have been admitted to a hospital or home for long term care; only one third would have been expected to continue to live in their own homes.

The results showed that community care:

- Halved the probability of death, halved the probability of entering an institution and doubled the probability of continuing to live in their own home
- Improved the perceptions of surviving clients of their state of wellbeing
- Improved performance in activities of daily living
- Improved the quality of care
- Reduced average costs to the social service departments without imposing additional costs to the health service
- Relieved the burden on carers.

Care management therefore had some experimental basis to suggest it would work. The benefits expected from care management have been set out in practice guidance around implementation of the legislation.[5,8] These are:

- To tailor services to individual requirements
- A commitment to individual care planning, to be shared with the user
- A division between assessment and service provision
- A more responsive service

- A wider choice of services across the statutory and independent sectors
- More involvement of users and carers
- Improved representation and advocacy for users and carers, including better complaints procedures
- Improved response to disadvantaged individuals including disabled people, people from black and minority ethnic communities, and female carers
- To have greater continuity of care and greater accountability to users and carers
- To have better integration of services, both within and between agencies.

The question is whether the new arrangements have actually delivered these benefits to the care of elderly people.

The role of the primary care team

The role of health service professionals, including general practitioners, is critical to the process. Health service staff involved in giving care to elderly people, such as district nurses or health visitors, may pick up changing needs which need to be fed back into the care management process. They also need to be fully aware of the care package being provided and who is the key worker.

The general practitioner is often the person to whom older people or their families turn if they have problems. People do not define their problems as "health" or "social", they present with their problem which may or may not seem "appropriate" to the professional. General practitioners will thus often be the first people to pick up on problems experienced by elderly people living in the community.

In an average general practitioner's list size of 2000 patients, 120 will be over 75, of whom 40 will have a severe physical disability and 12 will be in residential or nursing homes; 12 people aged 60–74 will have a severe physical disability. A shift of 20% from institutional care would result in two or three more people over 75 on the doctor's list living in the community. The role of the general practitioner with the primary health care team is to provide primary medical care to this population and to enable the care management process to be effective when needed. The general

General practitioners should:

- Be aware of referral process to social services
- Know whom to contact
- Know the eligibility criteria for services
- Know the possible range of services
- Know the key worker for individual patients
- Know the care package provided to individual patients
- Monitor changing needs and foresee potential problems
- Be aware of risk
- Participate in joint training

practitioner may make an initial identification of needs and will then need to make a referral to the social services department. They need to know who to contact and to be clear about eligibility for services. They may be required to contribute to the needs assessment process by providing health information about a patient (with their consent) or doing a health assessment (the over 75s annual checks for elderly people could be a useful source of information). Referral for a specialist's opinion may be necessary. If a person is considering entering a residential or nursing home it is essential that a full medical assessment has taken place to ensure there is no reversible medical condition contributing to the patient's inability to live at home. This assessment may well involve seeking an opinion from a specialist in geriatric medicine or old age psychiatry. If a person is to enter a nursing home at public expense, then authorisation from the health authority is necessary in all but the most urgent cases, which will require an assurance that a medical assessment has taken place.

General practitioners need to be kept informed by the local social services about the procedure for accessing social care and whether a standard referral protocol with specific forms is in use. Also, general practitioner fund holders may be purchasers of community health services so will need to be involved in the care management process where these services are to be deployed for individual patients.

61

General practitioners should be consulted about the development of new referral and assessment procedures. They can also contribute to information and objectives to be included in the annual community care plan. General practitioner fund holders can prepare their own purchasing plans in line with the community care plan. Locality planning teams for social services, which involve health authority purchasers and general practitioner representatives, should be planning local social service provision for a defined area. The development of locality commissioning by health authorities involving general practitioners to purchase health care, which may eventually replace general practitioner fund holding, has the potential to bring together the planning and purchasing of local health and social service provision. It remains to be seen if better coordination will in fact be achieved.

General practitioners also need to be informed about hospital discharges and whether an assessment for community care has taken place in hospital and what services will be organised. They are key professionals in liaising with social services to try to ensure coordinated services for their patients which will fulfil their social and health needs. There are often liaison nurses in post who coordinate community nursing aspects of patient care on discharge.

There is, however, a dilemma for some general practitioners who may encourage older patients to enter residential and nursing homes in which they or colleagues have financial interests.

The responsiveness of social services to elderly people's needs varies across the country. Budgeting constraints, particularly in the metropolitan areas, may mean that it is difficult to access services, and there may be difficulties making a referral. Many general practitioners feel very frustrated by what they see as inadequate responses by social services. Often, a general practitioner is called in by the family when a situation has reached crisis point, with a demand that "something must be done" if the elderly person is perceived as being at risk. General practitioners' services provide immediate care, 24 hours a day, seven days a week, and doctors find it hard to understand why social services cannot also provide immediate responses. The concept of urgent may be interpreted differently by health practitioners and social workers, and this can be an area of conflict. One bad experience in working with social services may colour a general practitioner's attitude and expectations for the future, and lead her to generalise that there is a systematic failure by social services ever to do anything. These attitudes can make relationships difficult and may result in older people not being referred for appropriate services because "there is no point". This situation can be improved only by each service having a realistic awareness of the way the other works and a willingness to work collaboratively to solve problems. Adequate information exchange is essential, and joint training initiatives are helpful. Some practices have attached social workers, and this can foster good working relationships. If a deteriorating situation for an elderly person can be recognised before there is a crisis then a proper assessment and action can be implemented in a planned, coordinated way. General practitioners and social workers need to look ahead at potential problems and not just respond to the immediate. This is a different way of working from the usual responses to the heavy caseload which both general practitioners and social workers carry and is one of the many challenges to professionals working with elderly people.

The other members of the primary health care team will also be interacting with each other and with workers from other agencies. Good collaborative working skills and understanding of different roles need to be fostered to ensure the best possible care for older people.

What sort of social care can be provided?

The budget for community social services is controlled by the local authority within their allocation from central government and revenue from the council tax. Money has been transferred from central government funding for social security to local government to pay for elderly people entering residential or nursing homes who are eligible for public support. However, the budget is not ringfenced. Services can be provided by in-house employees of the local authority or may be contracted with the private or voluntary sector. One of the aims of legislation was to stimulate diversification of the private sector into new areas to provide more choice and availability of services to meet individual needs.

The individuals themselves may of course buy in private sector care if they pay for it themselves or they may receive care provided by the voluntary sector. Elderly people may need support in the activities of daily living, and the aim is to provide help in individual care packages to meet an individual's need.

There are sometimes conflicts about defining what is social care—purchased by the local authority—and what is health care—provided by the health service. An example of this is bathing or transfers in and out of bed; in some areas social services will provide this service, in other areas the health service. It is important that policies are clear between agencies so that the elderly person does not get caught in the middle with no service at all. The danger of cost shunting between agencies is clear.

The importance to the user is that health care is provided free at the point of delivery; social care may be charged for. Different social services have different charging policies, depending on what has happened in the past.

Social care can be provided for transfers, cooking and the provision of meals, help with household tasks, such as cleaning and laundry, shopping, etc, and other tasks which may come to light in the needs assessment. Care can be provided at home or outside the home—frail elderly people may get social support by attending a day centre, and this may also give a carer respite. Each local authority will have access to different providers of services.

The aim of the community care legislation was to provide imaginative and innovative responses to individual need, rather than to fit the person into the available services. It is therefore difficult to give a precise description of services provided through social services departments as these will vary. Most social services departments, however, will either provide or contract for the sorts of services listed below.[9]

Home care—The role of "home helps" is being expanded and changed, and home care workers now often give basic personal care which has in the past been supplied by nurses. Simple domestic tasks may now not be done (such as cleaning), and the elderly person will be encouraged to employ a private cleaner. Shopping, laundry, and collecting pensions can also be provided by home care workers. They may also prepare breakfasts or leave sandwiches for later in the day and provide help with washing and dressing. There is usually a charge for the services.

Meals—A cooked midday meal can be delivered to the patient's home by meals-on-wheels (which may be organised by the voluntary sector); the service may be supplied seven days a week. Frozen meals can also be delivered. There is a charge for the meals.

Housing adaptations—Stair lifts, grab rails, bathroom adaptations, widening doors for wheelchairs, etc, can be provided through social services, usually after an assessment by a community occupational therapist. These will be charged for, after a financial assessment, if the elderly person lives in his or her own home; some adaptations will be paid for all or in part by the housing department of the local authority if the property is rented from the council.

Equipment for daily living—If equipment is needed to promote independence and safety in the activities of daily living—for example, in dressing, using the toilet, cooking, reaching, and lifting—it may be supplied, usually on permanent loan. Again, an assessment by the community occupational therapist may be necessary. (Mobility aids, such as frames and walking sticks, are supplied by the health authority as are nursing aids, such as special mattresses, hoists, etc). Wheelchairs are supplied by the local wheelchair service; arrangements will vary from place to place.

Respite care—Relief for carers can be arranged to give a period of time off from the task of caring, varying from a few hours to several weeks. Sometimes an older person living alone may also be offered respite care to give them a break from the struggle of being independent if they are finding it hard to cope. Respite care can be offered through:

- Sitting service—Usually provided by volunteers (for example, Crossroads schemes) where a person comes into the home to sit with the older person, allowing the carer to go out for a few hours.
- Day centres—These may be organised by the voluntary sector or social services, and attendance is on one or more days a week. Transport is arranged and lunch is provided. There may be specialist day centres for mentally confused people or people from particular ethnic groups or for blind people. If elderly people are very disabled and have difficulty negotiating steps outside their house or their house is not wheelchair

accessible they may not be able to attend a day centre as transport is often not specialised and staff are not able to carry people in and out. There is usually a charge for day centres.

- Family placements—Some social services departments offer placements with a family for a short period of time, a sort of "foster care".

- Residential or nursing homes—Short breaks may be offered in either social service residential accommodation or in private residential and nursing homes. A regular commitment to residential care may be given, "rotating" care or "intermittent" care, for example, two weeks in every eight. A charge will be made for this after a financial assessment.

- Short holidays—Care may be offered in residential homes or special hotels in a holiday location, for example at the seaside, to give elderly people a holiday.

Residential and nursing home care—If a person is going to be publicly funded for a permanent placement in a residential or nursing home a full assessment of their need must have taken place through the care management process. If they are paying for themselves there is no requirement for an assessment (although admission to a local authority run residential home would still be done on need). A few residential homes are still run by social service departments (Part III homes) but most are in the private sector. Private residential homes must be registered with the social services department, who should monitor them to ensure the standard of care is adequate. Private nursing homes must be registered with the local health authority, who are responsible for monitoring standards. Social service departments will hold a list of private residential and nursing homes. Families and elderly people themselves choose the one they wish to apply for; social workers and health workers should not recommend any home in particular.

Communication aids—Telephones and alarm systems may be supplied by social services to vulnerable elderly people.

Housing repairs—This area is quite often neglected but may cause a lot of anxiety to elderly people. Social services will be involved only if adaptations are needed because of disability. "Care and repair" schemes may be partially funded by social services through joint finance initiatives, and there are renovation grants made by local housing departments.[10]

The above descriptions are to give an idea of the range of services which may be offered or contracted for by social services, but local variations will apply, and professionals working with older people need to be aware of local arrangements.

How is community care working?

One of the fundamental objectives of the NHS and Community Care Act 1990 was to provide a seamless service to users and carers with a corporate approach to community care by statutory and independent agencies.

Agencies have to negotiate specific agreements which specify respective areas of responsibility, which are detailed and explicit. Good communication systems, standardised referrals, and assessment schedules and sharing of information have to be developed.

Joint training of workers in all agencies is essential as professionals from different agencies will have differences of attitude and approach, which are inherent in the different organisational cultures.

Joint working between health, social services, voluntary, and private sector, on the production and implementation of the annual community care plan is mandatory. Working towards joint purchasing of services from a pooled budget between health and social services could be a pattern in the future but requires a level of trust and mutual understanding which may well take years to achieve. Formal interagency schemes have been set up in some areas, sometimes with designated workers drawn from two key agencies (usually health and social services) or sharing care tasks between professionally and vocationally qualified staff, in specially set up multidisciplinary teams for elderly people or by strengthening the primary care teams. Close working relationships can foster interagency understanding and knowledge and skills can be shared, but there is also a danger of professional isolation, and elderly people may be stigmatised if there are special teams dealing only with them. Professionals may not choose to work with just elderly people because of negative attitudes, and there may be a difficulties in recruiting high quality motivated staff.

The challenge of interagency working, when the agencies have different cultures, patterns of working, philosophies, and expectations, should not be underestimated. For instance, social services are directly accountable to local politicians elected in the area whereas the accountability of health purchasers is directly to central government, and many health providers are quasi autonomous bodies. Local politicians may have firm views as to charging policies and the delivery of services. If services are to be delivered to those in greater need, then this may mean services such as home helps may be withdrawn from those in lesser need; this may be appropriate in the light of needs assessment but may be politically unacceptable. There is evidence that interagency cooperation is improving, however, and that efforts are being made to provide responsive, seamless services.[11,12]

The main problem in providing effective community services is finance. The Audit Commission in 1996, evaluating the implementation of community care in England, found that financial issues dominate the agenda.[13] Most authorities are having to take action to keep control of expenditure. Spending on community care is 7% more than proposed by the government.

Financial commitments depend on the number of people receiving care, arrangements for meeting people's needs, and the cost of each episode of care. The number of people receiving care will in turn depend on the numbers seeking help and the eligibility criteria—there is wide variation between authorities and criteria are often complex and difficult to understand. One way to control expenditure is to tighten eligibility criteria thus cutting some people out of help altogether. Most authorities are managing to improve the mix of services by increasing home care and by increased targeting on the very dependent, with more hours per household. The price of local authority provision has often been found to be higher than services provided by the independent sector, charging policies are being introduced,[14] and charges to individuals are increasing, which may affect uptake of services. There are still some perverse financial incentives to encourage placement in residential care if the cost of intensive home care is too high. Cost ceilings for home care are being introduced in some authorities. Recent cases have gone to judicial review,[15] and it has been found that it is lawful to take into account available resources when deciding what care can be offered. (A woman had been receiving 24 hour care which could be most economically provided in a nursing home, and she was placed there.) It is not lawful, however, to take into account resources when determining the needs of disabled people. This judgment will be contested in the House of Lords.

One major aim of the new arrangements was to encourage more people to live at home with better provision of domiciliary care and to reduce the numbers of elderly people going into residential and nursing home care. There is some evidence that fewer people who are publicly funded are going into nursing homes and are being placed in residential homes after detailed assessment of need by health and social services professionals. The overall number of elderly people in private residential and nursing homes is still increasing, but the proportion with regard to the whole elderly population is reducing, and there has been an increase in domiciliary care and respite schemes.[16]

There have been examples of delays in hospital discharge of elderly people both to their own home and placement in residential or nursing homes. This has been a particular problem in some metropolitan areas, with delays in the process of assessment and shortage of finance in local authorities to fund placements and domiciliary packages of care. This has led to prolonged length of stay in some areas and a notorious decision by one hospital trust to refuse to admit patients aged over 75 because of the difficulties of discharging them.

Users and carers should be at the forefront of planning community care. Some progress has been made in achieving this aim, but much still remains to be done.[17]

Most evaluations of the new arrangements for community care have been around process not outcome, but more data are being collated, and only time will tell whether the arrangements are really delivering better care to elderly people.

The future

The major challenges to be faced in the implementation of community care are of local authority finance and the difficulties of interagency working, particularly between front line professional staff. The change in approach needed to assess need and not just provide existing services requires a lot of support and training. There are major ongoing training requirements for all staff, including general practitioners and hospital specialist staff: vocational training and Calman-type training for speciality registrars should cover the delivery of community care to elderly people.

The increased privatisation of care, with a need for adequate monitoring of standards, also presents challenges for the public sector. There is, as yet, little evidence that the private sector has diversified greatly to provide new services, although this may happen slowly. There are arguments against believing that the market is the best way to plan service provision, although this is the ideology underlying the legislation.

1 Department of Health and Social Security. *Public support for residential care: report of a joint central and local government working party* (Firth). London: DHSS, 1987.
2 Audit Commission. *Making a reality of community care.* London: HMSO, 1986.
3 Griffiths R. *Community care: agenda for action.* London: HMSO, 1988.
4 Department of Health and Social Security. *Caring for people. Community care in the next decade and beyond.* London: HMSO, 1989.
5 Department of Health Social Services Inspectorate, Scottish Office Social Work Services Group. *Care management and assessment: practitioners' guide.* London: HMSO, 1991.
6 Challis DJ, Davies BP. Long term care for the elderly: the community care scheme. *British Journal of Social Work* 1985;**15**:563–79.
7 Challis D, Chessum R, Chesterman J, *et al.* Community care for the frail elderly: an urban experiment. *British Journal of Social Work* 1988;**18** suppl:13–42.
8 Department of Health Social Services Inspectorate, Scottish Office, Social Work Services Group. *Care management and assessment: managers' guide.* London: HMSO, 1991.
9 Renwich D. Community care and social services. *BMJ* 1996;**313**:869–72.
10 Warklyn P. Homes and housing for elderly people. *BMJ* 1996;**313**:218–21.
11 Audit Commission. *Taking care: progress with community care.* London: HMSO, 1993.
12 Audit Commission. *Taking stock: progress with community care.* London: HMSO, 1994.
13 Audit Commission. *Balancing the care equation: progress with community care.* London: HMSO, 1996.
14 Findings Social Care Research. *The impact of charging policy on the lives of disabled people.* London: Joseph Rowntree Foundation, 1996:80.

15 Appeal Court. Gloucestershire County Council, Lancashire County Council, Lord Justices Hurst, Swinton-Thomas, Sir J. Balcombe. May 1996.
16 Chief Inspector. Social Services Inspectorate. *Progress through change. Annual report SS1.* London: HMSO, 1996.
17 Department of Health. *Information on community care post April 1993: the concerns of users and carers.* London: HMSO, 1994.

4 Community health services

After 50 years of exhortation and experimentation in team working in the NHS the Standing Medical and Nursing and Midwifery Advisory Committee was able to say in 1996,

> *All professionals in the health and social services should adopt a collaborative approach to working across organisational boundaries, so that services users and their informal carers receive help which is timely, well coordinated, effective and appropriate to their needs.*

The difficulties that different professional groups have in acting in the patient's interest are very evident in the care of older people in the community, where team working remains problematic partly because the professionals involved are engaged with the problems of aging by accidents of history.

Health policies that have evolved over years now shape the delivery of medical and nursing care to older people living in the community both through the variety of services that operate and through their interrelations. Changes in the NHS and social services over the years have not only affected doctors, nurses, and other clinical staff but have also altered the roles of many ancillary staff. As delivery of effective care depends on good multi-agency working it is important to understand how the structure has changed and the implications of these changes. The reforms of the NHS over the years have often improved certain problems and have exacerbated or created others.

From the inception of the NHS in 1948 there was a tripartite structure. The hospital sector included boards of governors of teaching hospitals and hospital management committees. Community services such as community nurses, environmental health, family planning clinics, and home helps worked under the auspices of local government. There were also separate executive councils governing general practitioners, dentists, and pharmacists. Each group was answerable to the secretary of state for social services. This general structure was maintained until 1974. During this period hospital consultants were the main power brokers. Most of the funding available was controlled by hospitals and the agenda for medical education and research was set by them. The services employed by local authorities were the poor relations in this structure; they suffered from a lack of both resources and vision for the part they might play, particularly in preventive health care. The emphasis in this model was on cure which did not fit very well with the pattern of morbidity and disease which had shifted from the "acute" to the "chronic". Another feature of the legislation was that under Part III of the 1948 National Assistance Act local government was obliged to provide residential accommodation which came to be known as "Part III Accommodation". This was provided for the "elderly or infirm" who did not require constant medical attention.

In the 1989 white paper *Caring for People* the distinction was made between health and social needs.[1] The purchaser–provider split, in which the units responsible for assessment of an individual's service requirements differ from those responsible for providing the services, has resulted from this legislation. Another aim of the paper was to develop a mixed economy of provision of domiciliary care. While this has been achieved in the provision of residential care, there is little growth (so far) in private sector provision of services to people remaining in their own homes.

The recent health–social services split has also created problems for delivery of services. There has traditionally been a large gulf between social workers and general practitioners; the two occupational groups have very different cultures (summarised by Huntington[2,3]—see box). Although there has been a shift in recent years, many of these differences persist. In reviewing these differences, Dickie and Iliffe noted that while staff in social services may have some idea of the content of medical training, general practitioners seem to have little understanding of the requirement for or content of social work training.[4]

73

Differences between general practice and social work
(adapted from Huntingdon)

General Practitioner	Social Worker
Older	Younger
More often men	More often women
Leads team	Team member
Faster timeframe of working	Slower timeframe of working
Well respected, old profession	Less well respected, newer profession
Medical needs considered first	Psychosocial needs considered first
Self employed, less bureaucratic	Employee, more bureaucratic

Another study examined the impact of the community care reforms on general practice in North Thames Region.[5] There were general concerns about a lack of information and consultation before the changes. Furthermore, most general practitioners and social services representatives who took part thought that the aims of improving quality and choice of community services had not been realised. Concerns were raised at the increasing number of older people who were remaining in their own homes, with a perceived reduction in provision of practical support.

After the split, some services that were formerly provided by community nursing services became the responsibility of social services. Help with bathing is a case in point; community nurses and social services assessors have to decide whether the bath is a "social need" or a "health need". This distinction is often not entirely clear but charging policies will differ depending on the decision made; social care is means tested whereas health care is free at the point of delivery. Admissions to nursing and residential homes are now guided by multidisciplinary team assessments though the final decision rests in large part with the social worker (see chapter 3).

Nursing

Until 1974, community nursing services were organised by local authorities. Nursing teams were usually based in centres, separate from other health professionals. District nursing sisters were usually experienced, former hospital ward sisters. Health visitors had to undertake further training but this was not mandatory for district nurses, although the Queen's Nursing Institution offered such a course. Since 1974 community nursing services have been the responsibility of the district health authorities. Many other changes were taking place in primary health care in the 1970s. There was a move towards situating multidisciplinary teams in health centres; and the idea of the primary health care team was being taken more seriously. There was also a move within general practice towards group rather than single handed practices. After the Cumberledge report in 1986, many authorities attempted to implement "neighbourhood nursing", targeting a population within a geographically defined area. This can, particularly in densely populated areas, create yet another non-coterminous boundary. However, this shift was mirrored by moves within social services and housing departments towards localities. The perceived boundaries of a neighbourhood change with time because of local events such as population migration and structural changes. The advantage of using a neighbourhood as an operational unit, however, is that there will already be some infrastructure, including pre-existing local networks and a "sense of community".

Community nursing staff include district nursing sisters or charge nurses and their teams, health visitors, and school nurses, and they are usually based in health authority clinics or health centres. There may also be community midwives, and in some rural areas one person, the "triple duty nurse", combines the roles of district nurse, health visitor, and midwife. With the introduction and expansion of fundholding in general practice some community nurses are directly employed by general practitioners.

District nurses

District nurses provide nursing care to people in their own homes. In Britain, this was formally set up in Liverpool in 1859 and was followed by the founding of *The Queen's Institute* in 1889. Despite such early Victorian origins, district nursing continued to be dominated by voluntary associations until the 1950s. After the NHS Act in 1946, local authorities were obliged to provide a free home nursing service, though they could continue to use voluntary associations. Many authorities appointed a Queen's Institute trained nurse as superintendent thus creating a link with the institute. A working party was set up in 1955 to examine the issue of national training standards. After this a four month training for district nurses was introduced nationally. This was against the wishes of the Queen's Institute, which ran a six month training course and advocated this as an appropriate training period. The influence of the institute continued in a diluted form until the 1974 NHS reorganisation which followed the Briggs report. There have been several changes to district nurse training since then in terms of admission criteria, course content, and length of training. Most courses last an academic year and now take place in universities; places are purchased by health authorities and staff are seconded, often with a formal agreement that they will work for the same authority for a minimum length of time after training.

With skill-mix revisions in recent years, the district nursing team is likely to be made up of a sister or charge nurse who is a registered nurse with a certificate in district nursing and other trained nurses employed on D, E, or F grades. The grade on which the nurse is employed will not necessarily reflect his or her qualifications or experience very accurately; it is more likely to depend on the amount of money available and the predetermined skill-mix for the team.

The increased throughput of patients in the secondary sector has meant that patients are often discharged at an earlier stage in their recovery and are more likely to need community nursing and medical input to their care. District nursing sisters or charge nurses have always had a predominantly elderly caseload because of higher levels of morbidity in this age group. Many have become involved in the annual "75 and over" health checks, and there is some evidence from a national evaluation of the checks that this involvement will increase.[2] In many areas the standard assessment form used by district nurses already provides a fairly comprehensive assessment tool (see box).

A care plan would be made based on this assessment to deal with any problems identified. This may include referral to other agencies for further assessment or for specific aids or appliances.

Unqualified nursing staff

Auxiliary nursing staff who do not hold a full nursing qualification may work under the supervision of the district nurse. They are

> ## A "typical" assessment form would include:
>
> Reason for referral
> Basic demographic details
> Lifestyle factors
> Functional ability
> Mental state
> Continence
> Medication use
> Availability of carers
> Use of other services

often now called "health care assistants" or "patient aides"; there can be considerable overlap in their role with that of home care assistants. They may have undergone some NVQ/SVQ training and will deliver basic nursing care and carry out a limited range of tasks according to the nursing care plan. There has been some controversy over some of the tasks they can carry out, such as measuring blood pressure; until very recently, only nurses who were trained or in training were allowed to do this. At a time when many newly qualified nurses face unemployment the development of this role is threatening, at least to some, and is seen purely as a cost cutting exercise. Some commentators have argued, however, that if used properly the health care assistant can allow qualified staff to use their time more effectively in delivery of quality patient care.[1]

Home helps and home care assistants

Home helps and home care assistants are provided through social services. Referrals are passed on to the home care organiser, who makes an assessment of the individual's needs. This includes a financial assessment as services are charged to the client. There is evidence that clients regard this financial assessment as an unacceptable intrusion and that many of the organisers feel uncomfortable carrying it out.[6]

The role of the traditional home help is to ensure that there is food in the home and to carry out those basic household tasks which the client is unable to do. There have always been restrictions around some tasks such as changing curtains and washing windows, mainly because of risk of injury while climbing ladders. This may be justifiable in the "employer-employee" context of health and safety at work, but it can often upset the client if their own standards are not being maintained. Clients are usually advised to make their own arrangements and pay for these services. Those in receipt of attendance allowance are expected to use this money for this purpose. The limited time available and competing priorities may compromise standards. If a client or patient centred approach is to be adopted, however, these issues will have to be resolved.

More recently home helps have taken on an extended role, and many now provide services such as the "social bath". Their official title differs between areas, often they are known as home care assistants; this distinction is made not least because there is often a pay differential. The situation is further complicated by the fact that many staff combine both roles.

One evaluation of home help services for older people in Scotland indicated that there had been a shift from the traditional role of carrying out household and cleaning tasks on weekday mornings to including more personal care and some evening and weekend work.[7] One of the recommendations of this report was that local authorities should provide, either directly or via independent providers, assistance with tasks such as window cleaning, curtain changing, and spring cleaning.

This shift into more personal care has opened up some problematic areas for both staff and clients or patients. Administration of medication is often expected of home helps; however, there are no guidelines on this and it is a matter which causes concern as home helps are usually not trained or expected to know about drug interactions or adverse reactions and are therefore less likely than trained staff to identify these. One study in Derbyshire indicated that 17% of regular clients required some help with use of medication and that more of this was asked of home care aides than of the traditional home helps.[8] The main help required was with opening packages and bottles and reminding clients to take their medication. There were also substantial numbers requiring administration of eye, ear, and nose drops and of suppositories and pessaries. In some cases arrangements are made between general practitioners and local pharmacists to dispense medication in special dispenser packs.[9] District nurses no longer organise weekly dispenser boxes of medication after the United Kingdom Central Council (UKCC) recommendations, but community pharmacists can do this, leaving the daily administration to the patient or the home help, or both.

The involvement of home care assistants in the care of terminally ill patients also presents some difficulties. Lack of medical and nursing knowledge may place them and the patient in an unsafe position. Dealing with relatives around the time of death can also be difficult, especially for those who lack training and experience in this. There is also evidence that clients of home helps have high rates of depressive illness. This too can present problems for people without specific training or experience. A general lack of understanding may mean that the client or patient is not referred appropriately or quickly enough. There is already evidence that even when depression is diagnosed by general practitioners it is untreated or undertreated.[10]

Several issues have arisen with the apparent shift from household to personal assistance. Clients may have to choose between these as their allocated contact time is restricted.[11] There is some evidence that clients prefer to deal with their own personal care and like household tasks to be carried out by a home help. It could be argued that this only reflects expectations of the service: older people have grown up with the idea that the home help carries out household tasks and that personal care is part of the nurse's role. The main reasons given by the clients, however, were that many household tasks are completely impossible whereas, by taking their time, clients could manage personal hygiene and dressing. This social-health dichotomy and realignment is further complicated by overlap in the roles of the health care and home care assistants.

It is clear that there is a considerable overlap between the work done by health care assistants or auxiliary nurses employed by health services and home care assistants employed by social services. Competing professional identities may work against provision of a seamless service. Is one way out of this problem to create a new kind of worker?

The new National Vocational Qualifications, which are accredited by the National Council for Vocational Qualifications (NCVQ; SCOTVEC in Scotland awarding the SVQ) were established in 1986 and can be used to train generic care workers for provision of services to older people. Competencies can be measured in the occupational areas of *"providing health, social care and proactive services"*. NVQs and SVQs can be obtained by completing a portfolio of competencies and part of the training will be delivered in the work place, usually with some support from local further education colleges.

Using the NVQ/SVQ framework to develop a generic elderly person's care worker may be one way of bridging the health–social care divide. As these workers are not professionally qualified, problems around professional ownership may persist. Contractual problems are also likely as in the current system they will be employed either by the NHS or social services. The main exception to this is where they are employed by using some sort of venture capital for a specific (usually time limited) project. Unqualified staff are already used in the 75 and over health checks, however, and the ongoing MRC trial is comparing their effectiveness with that of trained nurses. There is also some evidence that where home care assistants and health care assistants are working closely, for example when patients need augmented community services such as "hospital at home", a certain amount of skill transfer takes place.

Health visitors

The earliest health visitors in Britain were nominally employed as women sanitary inspectors, and the first of these appointments was in Glasgow in 1870. After the Factory and Workshops Act of 1891 such appointments became more widespread throughout the country, and in 1904 an interdepartmental committee called for national provision of a health visiting service. There was no association with the care of the sick, and there were no training requirements at this time, the emphasis was on middle class women who visited working class families and advised on child welfare. The use of volunteers for this role was usual at this time and persisted in some areas such as Oxford until the 1930s. In 1916 the Local Government Board recommended that health visitors should have two of the following: a midwifery certificate, a recognised nurse training, or a certificate from the Royal Sanitary Institution. Maternity and child welfare services benefited from the First World War, and the number of health visitors employed by local authorities rose dramatically during this time. In 1919 the Ministry of Health advocated two routes to certification for health visitors: a two year training course for candidates with no previous training or a one year course for trained nurses, graduates, and women with three years' experience of health visiting. In 1962 a new Council for the Training of Health Visitors replaced the Royal Sanitary Institution as the governing body for health visiting. Health visitor training is now conducted in universities and takes one year, after nursing training and at least two years' nursing experience.

Although health visitors are trained to deal with individuals and families "from the cradle to the grave", in recent years their role (with some exceptions) has focused exclusively on preschool children and their families. This raises some problems around the involvement of health visitors in the care of elderly people; most of them have little practical experience of this because of their statutory obligations to assess the under fives and their increasing involvement in child abuse cases and "dysfunctional" families. Many of the staff employed as health visitors have deliberately taken on this role because they wanted to work with young children and families; to impose on them a universal obligation of assessment of elderly people may not work. There is evidence, however, that where health visitors are employed with a specific elderly health remit they make a very useful contribution and are valued very highly.

Practice nurses

Since 1990 the number of practice nurses has risen dramatically, corresponding with changes in the general practitioner contract. A national census conducted in 1993 indicated that there were 15 183 practice nurses in England and Wales, representing 9400 whole time equivalent posts.[6] Although only 14% of them hold a formal community nursing qualification, more than half make domiciliary visits, particularly to carry out 75 and over assessments and to give flu vaccinations. Most (80%) practice nurses are involved in running clinics for the management of chronic diseases such as diabetes, hypertension, and asthma.

There has also been a sharp rise in nurse practitioners, some of whom have undertaken a course at the Institute of Advanced Nursing Education, which is part of the Royal College of Nursing.

Others are practitioners who by virtue of their experience in certain clinical fields have been appointed at this level. The latter follow in the tradition of the experienced ward sister or charge nurse, and this seems more in keeping with the original vision of the clinical regrading exercise of the 1980s, which sought to pay nurses adequately for their clinical expertise to retain them in clinical rather than managerial roles. The longest standing examples of specialist nursing roles like this in the community are: diabetic liaison sisters, who liaise between the hospital and the community and provide high level clinical input and support to diabetic patients; and paediatric community teams, which were established long before general hospital at home services became innovative practice in the United Kingdom. There is, however, no consensus within nursing over what constitutes a nurse practitioner, and some argue that it is no more than the experienced sister or charge nurse is doing anyway. The UKCC has not yet reached a decision on what constitutes a nurse practitioner or how to record this qualification; this is currently under review.

Occupational therapists

Occupational therapy services are provided by both health and social services, and they have an important role in rehabilitation and assessment of the safety of people's home environments. They provide aids and arrange for adaptations required in the home to enable people to live as independently as possible. Typically, they assess the suitability of the home environment for the patient or client concerned. This includes looking at the height of various household fitments and furnishings, such as chairs, beds, toilet seats, kitchen worktops, and they provide aids and adaptations to compensate for needs identified. They also provide aids to assist with "difficult" dressing tasks such as fastening buttons and putting on stockings. If independent feeding and eating is a problem for the patient the occupational therapist can provide different types of cutlery and dishes and mats to stop dishes sliding. Meeting identified needs depends on availability and access to the appropriate aids, and there are resource implications for this provision. This can present problems particularly where major adaptations, such as altering doors and doorways for wheelchair access and fitting showers with seats, are required. It is their role, with its focus on functional ability, which appears to span most closely the divide between health and social care, although such a role is more apparent in specialist "outreach" services than in primary care teams.

The overlap between health and social care inherent in the work of occupational therapists, however, contains a risk as well as an opportunity. Clinicians may favour less active treatment and more palliative care for older people with disease (see chapter 1), adopting a prosthetic approach that substitutes for lost skills and restores autonomy but not independence. Occupational therapists can become the technicians of this prosthetic approach, and if they are working with social services at some distance from a therapeutic clinical approach that emphasises the patient's future potential and the reacquisition of skills, they may unwittingly decrease their client's autonomy and independence.[12]

Other services

The services offered to well elderly people by chiropodists, opticians, and dentists are of vital importance in maintaining their functional ability and health status.

Eye care

The General Household Survey data from 1991–4 suggest that around a third of the over 65s have an annual eye test. Routine free eye testing was abolished in April 1989, and this has provoked some protest. People receiving Income Support or Supplementary Benefit are still entitled to have free tests and vouchers towards new spectacles. The cost of spectacles, however, invariably outweighs the value of the vouchers, placing a financial burden on the individual. The commonest causes of visual deterioration in the United Kingdom are macular degeneration, glaucoma, and cataract. Apart from correcting refractive errors, there is real concern that glaucoma will go unobserved and untreated until it is too late. One study which investigated the referral rate for glaucoma after the introduction of fees for sight tests showed a reduction of nearly a fifth compared with rates in earlier years.[13] Analysis of the survey data suggests that the uptake declined initially and then rose again, though the peak uptake is in the 50–55 year old age group. The incidence of glaucoma increases dramatically at 65 years and over, yet only a third of this age group have regular eye tests. As with many other preventive health initiatives, there is also a social class difference: of the uptake 40–50% are in social class I whereas only 20% are in social class V.

Chiropody services

Chiropodists offering NHS services in the community usually run clinics in a health centre and also undertake domiciliary visits. The main problems treated are foot ulcers; nail problems; corns; rheumatoid foot; and mechanical problems. Patients with diabetes mellitus, peripheral neuropathy or peripheral vascular disease are regarded as "high risk" and are prioritised. Referrals to chiropody services increased dramatically after the introduction of the 75 and over checks by general practitioners. In those practices which have monitored referral rates, however, it seems that the referral rates stabilised after the first year of the checks.

Dentistry

Poor oral hygiene and age related changes to saliva production, alveolar bone atrophy, and epithelial atrophy of the mucous membranes contribute to periodontal disease, which in turn is the major reason for tooth extractions in older people. Badly fitting dentures cause poor speech and can lead to poor nutrition. Many older people have very few of their own teeth and need good dental services. Apart from general dental practitioners, there are also community dental services, which mostly look after "special needs" groups but can also provide domiciliary dental care for people who are housebound.

General dental practitioners have provided primary dental care within the NHS since it began in 1948. Unlike other NHS services, however, dental treatment ceased to be "free at the point of delivery" in 1950. Charges to patients were introduced particularly to reduce the NHS costs for dentures; initially these were the only items to incur copayment. Over the years since then charges have gradually crept in on most items. The fees to dentists and charges for items are reviewed annually. In 1990 the dental contract introduced a "continuing care" aspect to dentists by rewarding them for preventive work as well as for specific treatments. This meant that a dentist's income was partially dependent on having a list of registered patients and resulted in the budget being overspent and, as a result, the 1991 contract linked pay increases to productivity. The ensuing conflict between the government and the profession led to the Bloomfield review of dental remuneration in 1992. In the meantime dentists, particularly in London and the south east, have increasingly moved towards providing private services and many of the health insurance companies in Britain now offer private dental insurance. The net effect of this is not in the spirit of good, preventive primary care; appropriate dental care may not be readily available to those in lower socioeconomic groups who are likely to have higher levels of disease. Although people on income support and those who qualify for low income entitlement (with certificate AG2) are exempt from charges, they may have difficulty finding a dentist carrying out NHS work.

Multidisciplinary working

Many health care staff are involved in the care of older people in the community. The interprofessional relationships between different categories of staff can be difficult, and the interface with other agencies can be problematic.

Multidisciplinary and interagency working takes time to set up and requires commitment from the individuals involved. It is, however, essential in the delivery of care to older people. Although the concept of the primary health care team has been around for many years, the reality of working in the primary health care setting is that teams do not always function well, with individual members having their own competing priorities. Three broad types of primary care team can be observed (see box on p. 86).

Many of the examples of good functional and full team working around the care of older people reported in the literature are pilot projects, often set up in areas with especially high proportions of older people or in response to some crisis. Although this means that not all the methods and findings will be generalisable, some lessons can be learned, especially about obstacles to team development (see box on p. 87). A common aim is one criterion for successful working. Appointing a key worker for the individual patient is another feature of good team working. Clarity about the roles of each of the team members also contributes to success as do clear lines of communication.

Primary health care teams

(1) Patient centred or "essential" teams, including only those immediately involved in care planning and delivery

(2) Task centred, "functional" teams where different professionals with overlapping caseloads meet to review and coordinate their work

(3) Organisation centred "full" teams which have a strategic planning and development remit.

Source: *In the patient's interests: multi-professional working across organisational boundaries.* A report of the Standing Medical and Nursing Advisory Committees. Department of Health, 1996.

General practice or primary care?

The term "primary health care" is often used interchangeably with "general practice" by both policy makers and general practitioners, and the shift from the acute to primary care services has focused very much on general practice. As most of the population are registered with a family doctor this approach can be justified to some extent. While this is entirely appropriate for the provision of medical services, however, there is the inherent danger of taking too narrow a perspective on health. The gatekeeping role of the general practitioner has been widely defended, particularly in controlling access to secondary medical services, where it acts as a barrier to consumerism. It can also act as a barrier to patients who do not know the system, however, and have health needs which could be better dealt with by another member of the team. It also means that those patients need an appointment with the general practitioner first and then have to make another appointment to see someone else. Apart from being an inefficient use of time for both doctor and patient, it can cause transport problems for older people who may rely on the good will of friends or family or may have to use up more of their limited taxicard or "Dial a Ride" allocation. The central role of the general practitioner may not always be appropriate in team care for older people, although the gatekeeper tradition is reinforced by current changes towards fundholding and a primary care led service.

Sixteen obstacles to teamworking with older people

(1) No coordinated long term strategy for meeting needs
(2) Insufficient funds
(3) Disagreement over financial responsibility
(4) Competition between professionals or agencies to provide the same or similar service
(5) Lack of clarity about professionals' functions
(6) Short term planning done in isolation from other team members
(7) Poor communication between staff
(8) Unclear referral and assessment procedures
(9) Inadequate or overbureaucratic administration
(10) Local population falls within different geographic or administrative boundaries
(11) Different agencies or professionals situated a long way apart
(12) Staff inadequately trained and supported
(13) Different professional cultures, methods of working, resources, and organisation
(14) Mutual stereotyping of different professional groups (usually unflattering)
(15) Defensiveness among professionals—"turf wars" and "tribalism"
(16) Insufficient stability and continuity in structures and staff

Practitioners in all disciplines could usefully think about their work with older people in terms of basic principles of good practice.

The nursing contribution

Although there have been many "models of nursing" proposed in recent years, the "nursing process" for all its limitations may be a basis for health assessment among older people. The nursing process involves assessment, planning care, implementation of care, and evaluation. As part of this it is essential that clear care plans are made and that the care given is recorded. This should be a cyclical process so that after evaluation reassessment is made leading to a new care plan, etc. A holistic approach to care is

87

Good practice in team working with older people

- The patient's dealings with health and social services should be as simple and uncomplicated as possible
- Patients should be involved in care planning
- The professional coordinating care for any patient should be known and accessible to them and to their carers
- Continuity of care should be preserved by agreement about roles and responsibilities between professionals and disciplines
- Duplication of professional effort should be avoided
- Care should be appropriate to need, with timely specialist involvement

---

encouraged, taking the patient's preferences and usual lifestyle patterns into account. While the constraints of the hospital setting often mean that only lip service is paid to some of these aspects, they can usually be more readily accommodated in the patient's home. It can be seen that the nursing process is very similar to the care management approach, and this similarity may contribute to more integrated working.

The Macmillan Cancer Relief Fund has audit criteria for assessing teamwork that could be applied to all primary care teams working with older people.

A patient centred approach is not without risk to older people in the present climate. In attempting to achieve patient centred care there is the danger of swinging from "paternalistic" to "consumerist" care, in which attributes of autonomy and choice are assumed to exist for all patients even when there is clear evidence of dependence and lack of choice in their lives. The precision needed to strike a balance between patient autonomy, involvement, and "centredness", and good care for vulnerable people necessitates the involvement of professionals who can make and defend the judgments they make with and about individuals. The language shift from patient to client, adopted by many health and social services professionals in recent years, has largely resulted from criticism of the paternalistic doctor or nurse–patient paradigm, but, as we argued in the introduction to this book, it loses the

---

Macmillan audit criteria for assessing teamwork

(1) Systems for referral to a comprehensive range of services are in place and understood

(2) Mechanisms for liaison between disciplines exist and are used

(3) Staff demonstrate awareness of differing roles, relationships, and responsibilities

(4) Mechanisms for monitoring team performance exist and are used

(5) Systems to inform patients and carers about the range of services and skills available exist

(6) Arrangements for liaison between patients and services are established

---

original meaning of "suffering" and reduces relationships to transactions.

New models of care

Some pilot projects to develop multidisciplinary and interagency working have yielded important lessons. It remains to be seen whether these models can be exported to other locations, but we present two that we think are likely to be particularly important examples for future service development.

Community care projects

The Community Care project in Canterbury was a collaborative venture between the county council and an academic social services research unit. It was set up in the 1970s and was designed to enable frail older people to remain in their own homes. Clients accepted onto this scheme were assessed as being eligible for admission to residential care. The main project workers were experienced social workers, and they were given a decentralised budget for the project. This gave them some flexibility in the types and quantities of services which they could provide, above and beyond existing statutory services. The "helpers" recruited to the scheme were matched carefully with the clients in terms of shared interests, compatibility, skills, and proximity. This seemed to be an important factor in maintaining good client–helper relationships. Payments made to helpers varied with the task and time involved. In the recruitment process the helper's commitment to helping was of primary importance and financial remuneration was secondary. The help given was mainly assistance with washing and dressing, meal provision, and shopping. The relationships which developed, however, seemed more like becoming an honorary family member, with helpers arranging some trips and visits outside the home for clients. The benefits to clients were apparent from an early stage in the project,[14] further evaluation confirmed these preliminary findings and also indicated that there may be cost benefits over institutional care.[15] The two groups for whom it was most cost effective were: extremely dependent older people who were both mentally and physically frail and relatively isolated older people with non-psychotic psychiatric disorders.

The flexibility of the service offered through the Canterbury project depended on adequate resourcing of social care, and lack of that precondition remains the main problem for replication of this example. Nevertheless, efforts are underway to close the gap between social and primary care in many areas, with care managers working with primary care teams on problems encountered in primary care. Much of this new approach is theory, as yet untried and untested on any large scale, and much of it is based on research projects usually run by people with high abilities and high motivations, often with extra funding.

Those developing services must therefore be careful in how they approach such necessary innovation, even if adequate long term funding becomes secure. To ensure that the newly forming links between primary care and social services continue to grow innovators must carefully consider their development and the evaluation processes used to monitor innovation. We now know enough about the problems that arise in making social and medical care cohesive to map out a research and development agenda,[4] which should include:

- More controlled studies, including randomised trials of innovative approaches
- Careful consideration of standardised and comparable outcome measures, for example hospital admission rates and other uses of services

- Consideration of different models of service development, for example:

  - Using different members of the primary health care team as care managers
  - Full integration of social and medical care at local level
  - Wider decentralisation of social services for inner city areas

- Fostering joint education and training
- Collaboration between research agencies from both disciplines, with input from health and social care economists.

Social care of relatively ill and dependent older people in their homes leads directly to consideration of medical and nursing care for the same group. What complex or specialist clinical support is needed to match the complex or specialist social support offered in the Canterbury project? And what structures are able to deliver such clinical packages? The answer may be "Hospital at Home".

Hospital at Home services for older people

The first Hospital at Home in Britain began in 1978 in Peterborough and for many years it was the only successful scheme operating. Home based specialist care is particularly appropriate for older patients, who constitute most hospital inpatients, often find hospital admission disorientating and distressing, and are at risk of injury and infection in the hospital environment. With all the changes in the NHS and increasing pressure on resources, there has been great interest in developing more hospital at home services driven by a number of factors.

- The health service budget must provide advanced medical technology and new treatment possibilities for an aging population, and the potential cost savings of Hospital at Home services attract the interest of purchasers and providers.
- Policy pressure on managers in secondary care to transfer resources towards primary care is a significant factor in promoting the idea of Hospital at Home, especially in London after the Tomlinson recommendations.
- Regional differences in the lengths of stay for similar conditions have drawn attention to potential savings from earlier discharge supported by Hospital at Home services able to maintain standards of care.

91

In practice the apparent economic benefits of Hospital at Home services have not been realised, except perhaps for early postoperative discharge. Early discharge after hip replacement supported by a general Hospital at Home service can save resources, with an estimated six bed days and £720 saved per hip fracture if 40% of all those having hip replacements had access to Hospital at Home services.[16] Prevention of admission through use of a Hospital at Home service within the NHS has not yet been proved to save resources, although we suspect that this will be demonstrated in the future, especially if studies achieve a comprehensive review of all costs including direct and indirect costs to patients; costs to carers and their families; and total costs to health local authorities and voluntary agencies and the community at large.

Why have Hospital at Home schemes not been more successful in the United Kingdom? There seem to be several reasons:

● The pump-priming funding needed for setting up the service has not been available, and NHS managers have been reluctant to tolerate dual systems of inpatient and Hospital at Home care.
● Hospital at Home services may not function as a true substitution technology but as a new facility used by people who would otherwise have managed in other ways, without hospital admission. Lowering of general practitioner referral thresholds may contribute to this, especially when social care becomes rationed and less accessible.
● Resistance to change in the belief, held by professionals and patients alike, that ill people are always better off in hospital, reinforced by public suspicion of government intentions towards the NHS.
● Professionals have felt threatened by Hospital at Home schemes, both in terms of professional identity and job security as hospital resources are transferred to community services, and also by worries about increased workload (in community services) and more dependency in the case mix (in hospitals).
● The lack of a clear large randomised controlled trial to prove that Hospital at Home is more cost-effective, equally efficacious, or superior in its clinical outcomes and results in more satisfaction for patients.
● Four organisations with different structures and cultures and with a history of poor communication have interests in Hospital

at Home services: hospitals, general practitioners, community health trusts, and social service departments.

Most successful schemes around the world have been hospital based and run, which has a number of advantages, including:

- Contact with the hospital can be good, allowing problems to be solved quickly to the satisfaction of both the patient and professionals in the community
- Hospital staff are more likely to refer patients into a Hospital at Home scheme if it is seen as an extension of the hospital's own service
- There is potential for greater ownership among the doctors and nurses within the hospital concerned, especially in market driven types of health service, where Hospital at Home schemes seem more likely to thrive.

Even within the United Kingdom, the types of Hospital at Home care offered have varied enormously. A clear strategy needs to be developed as to which form this type of care should take so that if it were proved to work well and efficiently it could then be developed and grow from a sound base. At the moment the heterogeneity of the schemes and their small scale reduce their prospects of survival, but well informed purchasers can assess the potential of new and existing schemes if they take a systematic view of service development and functioning. The case for developing Hospital at Home as a form of "hospital outreach" seems strong to us, and experiments that test such alternatives to the Peterborough model of general practitioner dependent care should be conducted. Below we describe an apparently successful Hospital at Home service designed to avoid admission of ill, older people to inpatient wards, which has some features of a "ward in the community".

The future

Current developments in provision of social care and health service may be pushing us towards the creation of a generic care worker to provide a seamless service for older people, with relegation of the current range of professionals to support, education, specialist intervention, and supervisory roles. We will discuss this prospect in the concluding chapter. Hospital at Home services may expand to provide specialist medical and nursing care in the community,

The Waltham Forest Hospital at Home[17] was funded by London Implementation Zone money and became operational on 15 September 1994. It was developed specifically to provide an alternative to admission to acute hospital wards and in practice operated as a "ward in the community", even though it was not designed in that way. This was innovative in the United Kingdom at the time. Despite a very short lead in time to going operational and initial problems with recruitment of staff, the Waltham Forest scheme developed successfully. The team size and skill mix improved, as demonstrated by an increase in patient numbers and broadening of the case mix. The care offered combined input from a trained nurse and patient aide with support from physiotherapy and occupational therapy as necessary, with the general practitioner retaining clinical responsibility but in practice being involved only when considered necessary by the nursing team, which also had access to specialist medical advice. By June 1995, there had been 102 complete patient episodes. These patients were mostly elderly, with a large proportion over 79 years of age. Over 90% had been admitted as a result of falls or acute episodes or for rehabilitation. The average length of stay on the scheme was: six days for acute episodes; nine days for falls; and 10 days for rehabilitation. Nearly all patients remained in their own homes after being discharged from the service. The team size and skill mix permitted flexible responses to patient need, and there was evidence of tapering of care and skill transfer. Comparison with hospital inpatients in the evaluation suggested that this was a substitution service for care of elderly people and that the length of stay on the scheme compared favourably with the inpatient group.

especially if general practitioners loose their monopoly over the development of primary care services. And other initiatives like the Healthy Cities projects provide specific arenas for the public discussion of the needs of older people. If these changes proceed the legacy of fragmented services and underdevelopment in the care of older people in the community may be overcome.

1 Department of Health. *Caring for people*. London: Department of Health, 1989.
2 Huntington J. Time orientations in the collaboration of social workers and general practitioners. *Soc Sci Med* 1981;**15A**:203–11.

3 Huntington J. *Social work and general medical practice—collaboration or conflict?* London: George Allen and Unwin, 1991.
4 Dickie S, Iliffe S. Working together? A research and development agenda for social services and primary care. *Br Journ Hlth Care Man* 1996;2:258–62.
5 Lloyd M, Webb S, Singh S. *General practitioners and the community care reforms.* London: Department of General Practice and Primary Care, Royal Free Hospital School of Medicine, 1995.
6 Lankshear G, Giarchi GG. *Home care services: reasons for refusal; an exploratory study into the reasons for home care refusals recorded by Devon Social Services teams.* Plymouth: University of Plymouth, Faculty of Human Sciences, Community Research Centre, 1994.
7 Evaluation of home help services for older people. *Integrate News* 1996;58:9–10.
8 Goldstein R. Assisting elderly people with medication - the role of home carers. *Health Trends* 1993;25:135–9.
9 Bell S. Dispensing with dosage dangers. *Care Weekly* 1994;13 Jan:15.
10 MacDonald TM, McMahon AD, Reid IC, et al. Antidepressant drug use in primary care: a record linkage study in Tayside, Scotland. *BMJ* 1996;313: 860–1.
11 Chetwynd M, Howard M, Reith L, et al. A shift of focus. *Community Care* 1996;29 Feb:26–7.
12 MRC. The health of the UK's elderly people. London: Medical Research Council, 1994.
13 Laidlaw DAH, Bloom PA, Hughes AO, et al. The sight test fee: effect on ophthalmology referrals and rate of glaucoma detection. *BMJ* 1994;309:634–6.
14 Challis D, Davies B. A new approach to community care for the elderly. *British Journal of Social Work* 1980;10:1–18.
15 Challis D, Davies B. Long term care of the elderly: the community care scheme. *British Journal of Social Work* 1985;15:563–79.
16 Hollingworth W, Todd C, Parker M, et al. Cost analysis of early discharge after hip fracture. *BMJ* 1993; 307: 903–6.
17 Gould MM, Iliffe S. Hospital at home: a case study in service development. *Br J Health Care Management* 1995;1:809–12.

5 Screening in general practice

Research carried out in the 1950s and early 1960s indicated that there was considerable unmet need among older people in Britain. This work prompted study into ways of meeting the health care needs of older people, a task made more important by the aging of the population at the end of this century. This focus resulted in the introduction of an assessment programme for older people in the 1990 general practitioner contract.

The terms of service for general practitioners introduced in 1990 require members of primary health care teams to offer annual assessments of health to patients aged 75 and over,[1] with a number of broad headings to guide the assessment:

- Sensory function
- Mobility
- Mental condition
- Physical condition including continence
- Social environment
- Use of medication.

It was unclear what was intended when the contract for general practice was changed to include this obligation, but it was widely interpreted as a requirement to "screen" the 75 and over age group. While there has been extensive research into the possible benefits of regular screening of older populations, the introduction of the 75 and over checks provoked extensive debate because of the lack of conclusive evidence that routine screening was worthwhile.[2] Nor was there a consensus on the best methods for such screening, despite nearly 40 years of study.

Taylor and Buckley's review of assessment of older people summarised the state of the art just before the introduction of the 75 and over checks.[3] Early findings of massive unmet need had not been confirmed by later work, which showed that older people were no longer avoiding consultations with their doctors, that most illness was either known to the general practitioner or considered unimportant by the patient, and that non-consulters were mainly healthy. Social change, improvements in the population's health, and changes in health services had seemed to make screening for hidden disease among older people inappropriate. The hidden problem of later life in Britain in the last quarter of the twentieth century is not undiagnosed illness but loss of function that was either unrecognised or wrongly attributed to "normal aging".

The workshop that Taylor and Buckley reported on emphasised the need for functional assessment, and the need to evaluate the range of different approaches to assessment that had developed within primary care.[3] Their emphasis on functional assessment was echoed in the introduction of the 75 and over checks, but guidance on how to perform the checks was not available because the evaluations they called for did not happen. We shall return to this theme in this chapter.

Progress has been made in one aspect of assessment of older people in primary care through the development of two stage approaches in which a brief screen is used to identify possible "cases" who can be further assessed in depth.[4] Others have attempted to define more clearly the methods of assessment to be adopted.[5-8]

Different approaches have been advocated such as the "birthday card" reminders, health visitor assessments, volunteer assessment, and the use of "linkworkers" who coordinate services. In practice, a mixture of methods is often used, with respondents to a postal questionnaire or invitation being seen by a practice nurse who uses a checklist to assess health status, while non-responders and the housebound are reviewed by other workers, including doctors.

There have been some evaluations of the assessment of the 75 and over population since 1990, most of which have reported patchy uptake among general practitioners, many of whom doubt the value of the checks.[6] There are fears that those most enthusiastic

---

Approaches to assessment of older people's health

- Postal questionnaires and "birthday card" invitations to participate in screening
- Health visitor assessments
- Volunteer assessments
- Assessment by trained, generic workers (linkworkers) who liaise with general practice, community nursing, and social services
- "One stop shops" and assessment clinics in general practice
- Opportunistic screening by general practitioners or practice nurses

---

about having health checks are among the healthiest in the population (the worried well); and that those most in need of assessment are least likely to agree to having a check. Need itself is neither objective nor easily defined and the NHS management executive's definition as *the ability to benefit from effective health care* depends on that care being available. Most health promotion activities in general practice are already delegated to practice nurses, perhaps indicating perceived inappropriateness of involvement of general practitioners in this.

Research evidence

In the absence of a programme of evaluation of the wide range of projects reported by Taylor and Buckley what can we learn from the research literature? In the past 15 years there have been a number of randomised trials of screening programmes for older people, in the United Kingdom, Denmark, and the United States. Different trials used very different interventions and outcome measures, but there are some common features. A rise in morale among elderly people involved in screening programmes was frequently noted. Referrals to all agencies tended to increase, including to specialist medical care in some studies. The duration of inpatient stay fell in some studies, possibly through early intervention in disease processes. Inpatient rates could increase, however, through a greater use of respite care. Reduction in mortality did occur in some trials, perhaps for the same reason that inpatient stays declined, but not in all. Until recently, no trial has demonstrated an improvement in older people's functional ability, and general practitioner workload decreased only in situations where alternative services were organised to bypass existing primary care services. A meta-analysis of trials showed that home assessment was associated with reduced longer term mortality and higher likelihood of staying at home but had no measurable impact on functional ability[7].

Since the introduction of the 75 and over checks research has largely focused on implementation of the assessment procedures, showing variable involvement by general practitioners and no standardisation of methods. The review by the Manchester group revealed a tendency to delegate assessment to nurses, little or no interest in the assessment process in many practices, and a low priority for 75 and over checks among FHSA managers.[8] We shall also return to these themes in this chapter.

Primary care workers now face a number of problems in research, service development and policy formulation which need to be solved and which are summarised in the box overleaf.

Refocussing assessment of older people

The recent review of assessment of older people in the community commissioned by the NHS Executive[9] has shown that:

- A range of approaches to assessment of older people in the community is in use, and several different models of good practice with very different features exist
- The NHS administration is unable to identify many instances of assessment of older people, suggesting that the 75 and over checks remain a low priority for the local NHS or that general practitioners as a whole are not putting great time and effort into them, or both
- When assessment is undertaken, nurses have important but not necessarily leading parts, allowing an emphasis on functional assessment to emerge, although strong pressures for "medical" assessment (the detection of hidden disease) remains.

What development in the 75 and over checks should now occur? Two changes since 1990 are relevant here: the emergence of

We know	But ...
That descriptive studies show that screening yields significant amounts of unmet "need"	Patients and professionals do not necessarily do anything about identified need
That RCTs show that screening and intervention can reduce mortality, reduce inpatient stay, increase referral to all agencies, and increase patient satisfaction	There have been no cost-benefit (or even cost minimisation) studies of these interventions and no estimates of their utility to older peole and their families.
The RCTs have failed to show improvement in functional ability	Recent studies in the United States are showing improved IADL scores after intervention
That "at risk" group are very hard to identify, making targeted screening difficult to implement	Risk factors for increased service use, disability, and cognitive impairment are established, making a high risk approach possible
There is no consistency in approach in British general practice and no standardisation of screening techniques	Consistency and standardisation have been achieved (Tremlett's work) where leadership is given by health authorities
When assessment is done it is mostly delegated to practice nurses, who probably lack appropriate training	General practitioners are better placed to do opportunistic screening given the right brief instruments for detection of functional loss and available services to take remedial action

practice nurses as a large workforce within primary care; and the near universal computerisation of general practice. Not all practice nurses have a background in community nursing work, with experience of assessing functional ability, but many do. Not all general practitioners make appropriate use of their information technology systems to collect detailed information about their patients, but an increasing number do. In the next decade these two changes could combine to transform the approach to assessment of older people in the community from an unpopular chore of dubious value to a central component of primary care. Considerable effort and resources will be needed to achieve this change, particularly through training of practice nurses, but before this begins several issues need to be resolved.

Information about the implications of the workload from the annual assessment package became available to general practitioners only after its introduction, suggesting that cost-benefit analysis had not been performed in the contract's planning stages and that the evaluation of different schemes proposed by Taylor and Buckley[3] was not being done. Development and evaluation of new approaches was needed.

Similarly, morbidity and disability are prevalent well before 75, so that the choice of age for annual assessment is arbitrary and may not be the most appropriate given limited resources.[10] Vetter and colleagues have recently challenged the value of screening programmes beginning at 75, through re-analysis of data from an intervention trial that used health visitors.[11] Secondary analysis of data from a random sample of patients over the age of 74 involved in a study covering all the elements of the annual assessment of elderly people suggests that the 75 and over age group is not homogenous, that annual screening may be too often for some and too infrequent for others, and that different assessment methods might be needed at different ages. If comprehensive functional assessment is to become the core of care for older people, its components may need to be introduced before the age of 75 and applied in flexible ways.

Redefining assessment

The idea of assessment itself needs to be clarified. The uses of assessment of older people can be grouped under five headings: preventive screening; measuring severity and monitoring progress; audit of clinical work; creating a database for rational resource allocation; and basic research requiring population studies. At practice level the key questions are: Should the practice be screening its whole population of older people, and if so how?; Should staff concentrate on assessments with any particular groups of older patients, and if so which?; and Does assessment have a deeper meaning for clinical care, adding detail to the understanding that professionals have about specific patients? These questions cover population screening, case finding among those already in contact with the service, and assessment of patients to aid clinical management.

The ethical issues associated with each use of the term assessment demonstrate how problematic preventive screening is. To be ethically acceptable preventive screening of elderly people should be acceptable to the people themselves, have a validated process with sensitive and specific screening instruments, and identify remediable problems for which resources exist. In addition, the screening process should yield more benefits than dangers—particularly medicalisation of old age, overtreatment, and poor quality assessment—while preserving confidentiality.

Annual screening of the kind apparently required by the current general practitioner contract does not fulfil these criteria and logically should not be pursued in its present form. As Williams makes clear the form of assessment with the fewest ethical objections, most relevant to individuals and closest to usual practice, is comprehensive case management. This is essentially reactive, but a pro-active dimension appears when we consider its prerequisite—case finding.

Case finding and case management

Some of the problems experienced by older people are similarly prevalent at all ages above 75, including the proportions with signs of social isolation, regularly prescribed medication, and one or more major diagnoses recorded in the general practice record. These problems may well need regular review but logically this should occur after their onset and not at some arbitrary starting age. Nor is one system of review necessarily appropriate for them all. For example, it is difficult to see why social circumstances need to be reviewed annually rather than when they change, especially since for this population lone status may not be associated with higher morbidity[12] and lack of confiding relationships may not be associated with depression.[13]

Review of medication is an important task, given the extent of iatrogenesis, but annual assessment seems arbitrary and more frequent review may be appropriate and should anyway be a routine component of case management. In the North London study one in five of those aged 75 and over had no significant diagnoses recorded in the general practice record, and an even larger

Summary points

Assessment of older people can be . . .

- Preventive screening
- Measuring severity and monitoring progress
- Audit of clinical work
- Creating a database for rational resource allocation
- Basic research requiring population studies.

Preventive screening of elderly people should

- Encourage healthy aging
- Be acceptable to the people themselves
- Have a validated process with sensitive and specific screening instruments to identify remediable problems for which resources exist
- Yield more benefits than dangers
- Avoid:
  - Medicalisation of old age
  - Overtreatment
  - Poor quality assessment
- Preserve confidentiality

proportion had no regular medication prescribed.[14] Poor quality recording may account for some of this apparently healthy group, but general practitioners are rarely criticised for prescribing too little for their elderly patients, and the fact that between a fifth and a quarter were not receiving repeat medicines suggests that a considerable minority of very elderly people remain relatively well.

This does not mean that they lacked potentially remediable impairments. The prevalence of loss of hearing and vision among those aged 75 and over is high, and the well documented association between both hearing and vision loss and falls, together with the morbidity and mortality associated with falls, makes assessment of these senses an important task. In those aged 85 and over in the North London study five times as many people could not read the newspaper, even when wearing glasses, than among those aged 75-79. This may reflect not only untreatable macular degeneration

103

but also undetected and potentially treatable glaucoma, cataract, and retinopathy. Annual assessment of vision may well be appropriate for very elderly people, although it is arguable that it should be done by more skilled professionals than general practitioners, given the tendency of general practitioners to delay referral for glaucoma and their lack of accuracy in identifying retinopathy, even after training.

Hearing loss may similarly deserve regular assessment, both for those with hearing aids whose impairment cannot be assumed to be reduced and among those without aids. Although screening for hearing loss could usefully begin at a much earlier age, there remains considerable scope for ameliorating deafness in elderly people.[15] Again, the question arises, are general practitioners in the best position or sufficiently trained and equipped to assess hearing loss?

Continence

Urinary incontinence has a deleterious effect on quality of life, may be an important factor in the institutionalising of elderly people, and is expensive for health services, accounting for 2% of health care costs in the United States. Many women become incontinent after pregnancy; preventive measures such as training in pelvic floor exercises can help to avoid this. Intervention can improve the quality of life in a proportion of people suffering with urinary incontinence. Urinary incontinence is prevalent at all ages above 75 but not significantly more prevalent among those aged 80 and over.[15] Nearly a third of women in the 75–79 age band reported at least occasional urinary incontinence, suggesting that screening at 75 may be unnecessarily late. Among those aged 85 and over a higher proportion of men than women reported urinary incontinence, possibly reflecting the increased prevalence of advanced prostate disease.

Functional loss

Functional impairment and disability increase in prevalence with advancing age, but in the North London study almost all of those needing support services were in contact with them at the time of the study, and few requested extra help. Given the apparent capacity of social services to meet need in two London boroughs in the late 1980s, the new contract's requirement for general practitioners to screen for disability then seemed an unnecessary duplication of effort. The rationale for annual assessment of impairment in addition to ongoing clinical review and case management is difficult to see, but if such assessment is justified by the more recent contraction of social services it should be concentrated on the older age bands where reported impairment is greatest.

Psychiatric morbidity

Depression affects close to one in five elderly people but does not become more prevalent with increasing age and is mostly a "demoralisation syndrome" associated with disability. It is unclear how best to relieve this form of depression, although conventional medical treatments are effective with the small proportion of depressed elderly people with severe depression. Dementia, on the other hand, increases in prevalence significantly with age, affecting nearly a third of those aged 85 and over. No medical treatment is as yet effective in treating dementia of the common Alzheimer or multi-infarct types, but mobilisation of support services can significantly reduce carers' burden and psychological morbidity. Screening for significant psychiatric disorders among elderly people therefore seems to be a realistic option once uncertainties about the optimal management of depression are resolved.

While depression in later life is common, however, the ability of general practitioners and other primary care workers to identify it in their patients and respond effectively to it is limited. It might be appropriate to say that depression in later life is *underestimated, underdiagnosed, and undertreated.*

This situation calls out for change, which expert commentators over a decade ago suggested should be, *"to capitalise on the existing patterns of services used by the depressed elderly through which to improve the capacity of the primary health care network to recognise and treat these people"*.[16]

This is an argument against dedicated programmes and special teams, in favour of improving the performance of what we already possess—an elaborate network of general practice, community health services, and social care.

This finding is not unique. The Gospel Oak study, an intervention project led by psychiatrists that has been running for some years in a single ward in Camden, has failed to produce any reduction in the prevalence of depression in those aged 65 and over. Instead,

105

Depression in elderly people is

Underestimated because:

- Depressed people over the age of 65 are four times more likely to commit suicide than younger people
- Depression in later life is associated with high use of medical and social services
- Depression particularly affects those older people caring for others.

Underdiagnosed because:

- Community studies show underdocumenting of depression in medical records when compared with prevalence of depression.

Undertreated because:

- Not all of those who are diagnosed with severe depression are treated
- Depressed older people are likely to be treated for anxiety (or symptoms like pain) rather than with antidepressants or psychological treatments—even though the commonest drugs used for suicide by self poisoning among older people are painkillers and sleeping tablets or tranquillisers.

Research point

A study was designed to enhance the performance of general practitioners in detecting depression in older people by using a validated and relatively brief standard questionnaire—the 15 item geriatric depression score—in a small randomised controlled trial. The general practitioners were able to use the questionnaire in clinical practice, and they were able to detect twice as many people with depression when they used it compared with when they used only their own clinical judgment. But detection made no difference to their response, and there was no discernible difference between those identified by clinical judgment and those identified by the screening instrument in the prescribing of antidepressants or referrals to social services, to physicians for elderly people, or to old age psychiatrists.[17]

its research staff have noted consistent resistance among depressed people to the diagnosis of depression and reluctance to try or continue with antidepressant treatment. MacDonald noted in 1986 that, *"efforts to improve the recognition of depression in elderly patients by general practitioners will be wasted. Rather, examination of the management, related to outcome . . . would yield much of interest"*.[18]

In other words it is treatment, not perception or diagnosis, that matters in primary care. The problem in primary care is not that general practitioners do not treat depression because they do not see it but that they will not see that which they cannot treat. Efforts to make primary care staff into specialists by giving them summary forms of specialist expertise in the form of screening tests or guidelines may not be effective if they are not also given appropriate treatment options.

Why is late life depression such a problem for primary care? There seem to be two dimensions to the answer: depression in old age is far from homogenous in character, allowing the problem solving (rather than diagnostic) approach of general practice to focus on symptoms rather than underlying psychopathology; and limited access to the range of treatments that might be beneficial.

Most older people with depression fall into the "dysphoria" or "demoralisation syndrome" group, where the appropriateness of the clinical label is contested, often because the depression is associated with other problems, and where the effectiveness of treatments is unknown. Only a minority (about 3% of those aged 75 and over) have severe depression in which antidepressant treatment is known to be effective.

Depression in later life is characterised by variability of symptoms (and is sometimes dominated by anxiety), somatisation, high prevalence of depressive symptoms in the population, and its association with disability. Its identification is complicated by its overlap with other mental state disturbances (like dementia) and with organic mood syndromes (both endocrine and drug induced).

General practitioners faced with this complexity will tend to use pattern recognition and problem solving logic to try to help their patients. If the patterns learned by the general practitioner, either formally through education or informally through experience, are less complex than the reality some other problem will be "recognised"—anxiety, insomnia, or physical symptoms like back pain. Action will then be taken to solve these problems and

107

medication prescribed that may not be effective for the depressed person.

Enhancing pattern recognition, with a more complex understanding of depression in later life, may be appropriate and may justify the "Defeat Depression" campaigning approach to professional education and practice. If there are few, if any, effective treatments for most depressed older people, however, is there any point in becoming more perceptive? However, this is where community health services and social care may have better answers than medicine. Depression is likely to have social and historic origins in older people just as it does in younger adults, and social responses—through richer social networks, through opportunities for social activity, through work, through regular physical exercise—as well as psychological approaches may offer just the "treatments" that general practitioners lack.

Accessing these treatments requires knowledge of them, confidence that they have been tested and found effective, and close enough relationships with those that offer or guard them. These requirements may seem distant much of the time, especially as both general practice and social care diverge down increasingly commodified paths, but there is a strong sense of the importance of non-medical treatment options in general practice as the growth of counselling, rehabilitation, and alternative medicine in practice settings shows. The key to improving the quality of care for depressed older people in the community may lie with the idea of "networking", a notion that has entered the vocabulary of general practice in the past five years. Networking—as opposed to its medical rival, "referral"—is a social term implying dialogue and contact. Entering the network of social services, voluntary organisations, and community bodies like churches or other religious institutions may be the best that primary care workers can do to help depressed elderly people who are not responsive to medical treatments. The importance of networking is seen clearly when we consider screening for the second major psychiatric disorder of later life, dementia.

Dementia

The early signs of dementia are often missed by family members and professionals alike, and both groups may do little in response to the growing symptoms of dementia. This may not matter, as long as family members and professionals remain equally unaware. For example, interviews with the relatives of predominantly working class elderly people with early dementia in Cambridge suggested that most did not view the changes in their dementing relative as a matter of serious concern and saw loss of daily living skills as part of normal aging rather than as a symptom of illness.[19] In most instances the changes in the affected person had not been brought to the attention of their family doctor, possibly because of different social class attitudes to the role of the general practitioner with middle class families having a more social and less narrowly medical perception of general practitioners' functions.[20]

A similar study of relatives of elderly Italian people in whom a diagnosis of dementia had been reached during a hospital admission for an unrelated problem found three main reasons for delayed diagnosis: attribution of change to normal aging; respect for parents or grandparents; and negligible effect of the problem on family life and the family economy.[21] Even older people who have frequent contact with general practitioners may not report symptoms of forgetfulness or confusion. A community study in East London found only a minority of those aged 85 and over (with an annual consultation rate of seven) had consulted their general practitioner about memory or cognitive changes, although one in three experienced forgetfulness and one in six experienced confusion.[22]

If the early signs of dementia cause no major problems for those around the person whose cognitive function and everyday abilities are deteriorating, a diagnosis of dementia is not needed and is not made. We know that failure by general practitioners to diagnose dementia is common if medical records are compared with the results of population screening for cognitive impairment, and the diagnosis may be absent from the medical records of people with very advanced dementia. Some obstacle to documenting (rather than making) a diagnosis seems to operate because the ability of general practitioners to reach a diagnosis of dementia when prompted about particular cases in experimental studies is better than might be expected,[23] especially if guidelines for diagnosis are used. While some of the failure to document the diagnosis may reflect hurried and inconsistent record keeping, anecdotal evidence from carers and families suggests that there is also a real problem of recognition in everyday practice. Part of this problem of delayed diagnosis seems to lie with the clinician's own emotional response to the diagnosis and part with a limited conceptual framework for understanding dementia.

Interviews with Belgian general practitioners about their patients with dementia revealed that doctors (and patients) initially denied problems created by the dementing process, began the diagnostic process when the patient became a significant problem to others, and responded to the diagnosis—once made—with feelings of disbelief, of apprehension at the level of support that the family would require, of frustration at their own powerlessness, and of fear of dementia itself.[24] A similar process of being paralysed or overwhelmed by the complexities of the situation is described among nurses working with older people.

Practice points

Several factors seem to trigger the diagnosis of dementia:

- Disturbances in activities of daily living, including irregularities in use of medication in people who had previously been reliable in their use of prescribed medicines for long term problems

- Behavioural problems like expression of and action around paranoid ideas or hallucinations, which may cause major problems for family and neighbours

- Cognitive disturbances, with memory loss or orientation difficulties, so that bills are not paid, important things mislaid, or the person themselves becoming lost in familiar environments

- Crises—"revelatory moments"—like the sudden loss of support from a spouse who becomes acutely ill and is admitted to hospital or an intercurrent illness in the dementia sufferer, which adds acute confusion to the underlying but camouflaged chronic confusional state.

These diagnostic triggers and revelatory moments may result in urgent referrals to specialist services that may be perceived by other professionals as being "too late",[20] but can they be avoided by earlier diagnosis and more timely intervention within primary care?

Good practice

As general practice is a discipline that solves problems rather than reaches diagnoses, early detection of and earlier responses to dementia may not be feasible as long as the changes of dementia are contained within a family or social structure and wrongly attributed to normal aging. We know from experience, however, that there is sufficient mismatch between family perceptions and professional judgments about patients with symptoms of dementia to justify a more critical perspective and warrant investment of time and effort in promoting "good practice" in the recognition of dementia and in making responses to it. Four issues appear important in the development of such good practice in primary care: a population perspective on health care in later life; enhancement of diagnostic skills; application of the continuing care paradigm to dementia; and networking with appropriate social, voluntary and medical agencies.

Population perspective—The current 75 and over annual assessment of their health does allow a profile of the older population to be created and permits a systematic review of mental health, and this may allow earlier detection of unrecognised dementia and permit forward planning to minimise the impact of crises. If it is to be widely and effectively applied it will have to be seen as useful for patients and professionals alike, and this will require investment in training for primary care staff.

Enhanced diagnostic skills—The tendency to misdiagnose patients with physical frailty and functional psychiatric disorders as demented has been noted by general practitioners and may explain their tendency to overdiagnose the condition when prompted on a case by case basis.[23] None of the general practitioners in the Belgian study could give an operational definition of or accepted diagnostic criteria for dementia.[24] Nor did they include depression when discussing alternative diagnoses, but they did describe four of the key symptoms in the DSMIIIR criteria—disturbance in activities of daily living, activities of daily living behaviour change, memory loss, and disorientation—and emphasised the importance of the clinical picture and of informant histories.

111

Research points

Validated screening instruments, used either in population screening or in clinical encounters, seem to offer an alternative to enhanced clinical skills, but they are not widely used in general practice.

- In a study of general practitioners in Edinburgh only 14% used a standard cognitive function test[25]

- A second and wider survey found less than a quarter using such a test

- When general practitioners do use a standard instrument for detecting cognitive impairment on an opportunistic basis as a case finding tool (in a randomised controlled trial) their subsequent management and referral behaviour does not change[17]

A broader educational approach emphasising the complexity of the clinical picture in dementia, its evolution over time, the importance of informant histories, and the opportunities for useful responses may be more important than reliance on screening tests, and this approach has informed the production of a recent educational package (Alzheimer's Disease Society. *Dementia in the community: a management guide for general practitioners*. London, 1995).

Dementia and its emotional context—Broad educational approaches may not be helpful unless primary care professionals perceive the dementias as progressive neurological disorders that cannot be cured but for which a range of supportive responses still exists. The view that "nothing can be done" for advanced cancer would not be accepted today because so many options exist for relieving symptoms and helping the patient and others to overcome the problems of the disease. The same repertoire of responses is needed to overcome the therapeutic nihilism that dementia still provokes. Management strategies for medical, nursing, and social care workers will be accepted in primary care if they are seen to "work"—that is, relieve the patient's distress, reduce the burden on carers, restore a sense of effectiveness to professionals, and, whenever possible, avoid crises. Including advanced dementia as a condition suitable for a "continuing care" approach would signal such a change of perception.

Networking—Membership of a local network of services focused on early detection and support of people with dementia and their carers and rapid response at times of crisis seems essential if general practitioners are to optimise the care they give. Routes into such networks will vary, but old age psychiatrists may be in a good position to promote networking—for example, by promoting attachment of community psychiatric nurses to practices where they have been shown to provide high quality supportive care to dementia sufferers and their families as well as facilitating early diagnosis. Social service involvement is essential but, given the culture gap between social work and general practice and the limited resources available to social service departments, is perhaps the most problematic of all the tasks involved in network development.

A general practitioner or nurse who recognises the early symptoms of dementia in a patient but who then finds that the family do not perceive any serious change may be tempted to ignore their own knowledge and not document their findings. This is no longer justifiable because the suspicion of dementia will alter future consultations, cast urgent requests for help by family or neighbours in a different light, allow mobilisation of resources to be thought about in advance, even planned, and prepare primary care workers for discussion of diagnoses and responses when events reveal dementia as a problem. Initial suspicions may be wrong, of course, but they can be reviewed and checked by other team members only if they are recorded. That process of reviewing presupposes a pro-active approach to the problem of dementia among professionals who are expanding their knowledge base and repertoire of responses to a problem that will neither go away nor stay hidden for long.

Assessment: an alternative strategy

Firm recommendations on the most cost-effective method of assessing await the results of randomised trials, but the literature reviewed here favours more flexible forms of assessment than that

Comparison of assessment methods

Variable	Screening (of whole populations)	Case finding (among those seen)	Assessment (of those judged to be at risk or affected)
Sensory functions	No reliable brief screening test for hearing loss; Snellen chart widely used for visual loss but not reliable; screening for glaucoma not proved to be of benefit	No reliable brief screen test for hearing loss; red reflex test for cataract allows early detection and intervention improves quality of life; Intra-ocular pressure measurement in first degree relatives of patients with glaucoma, patients with hypertension, and those with symptoms	Referral for audiological testing unless possible in primary care setting; opticians can have an important role in primary assessment of eye disease
Mobility	Lachs 5 point scale too insensitive. No validated brief instrument available, little evidence of benefit from population screening	Use of simple activities of daily living scale justified in patients with cardiovascular, respiratory, and joint diseases to establish baseline dataset	Activities of daily living scale useful, Barthel appropriate only for most disabled. Community nurses, physiotherapists, and occupational therapists most experienced at assessment

Variable	Screening	Case finding	Assessment
Mental condition	No evidence of changes in professional behaviour and gain to patient as a consequence of population screening	Age related testing for cognitive impairment justified, as is use of a brief depression scale in patients with severe disabilities, insomnia, and anxiety	Clinical suspicion of change in mental state (in absence of acute confusion) justifies use of standard scales
Physical condition	No evidence of gain from comprehensive investigation in whole populations	Case finding for hypertension justified	Endocrine and haematological disorders relatively common, but best identified through response to symptoms
Continence	No evidence to support population screening	Urine testing allows symptoms to be elicited	Self report of symptoms seems sufficient to prompt appropriate examination
Social environment	No evidence to support population screening	No evidence yet to support case finding	No reliable measures suitable for primary care settings to caputure the complexity of social relationships
Medication use	Regular review of prescribing for the whole population of older people is possible with current information technology systems	Special attention to all older people receiving repeat prescriptions is appropriate	Inappropriate prescribing seems to be more of a problem than drug interactions

115

required by the new contract for general practitioners. We have tried to summarise these in the table on pp. 114–15.

Opportunistic case finding among mobile and relatively well people taking few, if any, prescribed medicines seems appropriate for most of the categories of the annual assessment where the low prevalence of most problems would make screening with home visits too costly. The high consultation rate of the elderly population makes opportunistic assessment feasible provided that assessment focuses on the commonly missed problems—psychiatric morbidity, urinary incontinence, and impairment of vision and hearing. Analysis of consultation patterns may help to identify those who are becoming disabled and in need of more detailed assessment.[26] This analysis could be initiated before the age of 75 and repeated perhaps three yearly until the age of 84 years or disability supervenes.

Very elderly people probably need a more intensive approach as will some particularly ill or disabled people of younger age. Annual assessment in those aged over 85 may be insufficient for the most disabled but probably should be the baseline service offered to all, even if they are currently well and managing to their own satisfaction, to anticipate problems and allow forward planning of services. With these groups the use of relatively complex instruments with good performance for dementia and depression would seem to be justified given the prevalence of mental ill health and the need to minimise reassessment of "false positive" cases. Disability can be investigated, if necessary by using more complex activities of daily living scales.

The Community Care Act

Are general practitioners best placed to make comprehensive assessments of both medical and functional needs of older people in the sense of having the skills and organisational framework for such activity? Certainly there is no tradition of this approach in general practice, except among a few enthusiasts, and the widespread delegation of assessment of elderly patients to nurses or even lay volunteers suggests that many general practitioners remain uncomfortable with the role imposed on them. Social service departments have a tradition of needs assessment that has been codified and formalised by the Community Care Act, with specific roles allocated to general practitioners in the assessment process. Giving general practitioners a specifically medical role in an assessment procedure initiated by social service workers seems more rational than elevating them to a leading role in assessment without suitable training.

The future

The failure of the current contract to make clear the purpose of annual assessment of elderly people hinders the development of cost-effective and patient friendly assessment protocols. If prevention of a severe disability like loss of mobility becomes possible then mass screening may be justified but only if intervention of proved benefit can be offered. If, however, improved management of medical and social problems is the main aim then assessment should be focused on the very elderly people, whose need is likely to be greater. At the present time the latter seems more appropriate than the former, and it would be sensible to rewrite the general practitioner contract to redefine assessment of elderly patients in this way.

The North American model of assessment by community based geriatric consultation teams may be applicable here. Such multidisciplinary assessments have been shown to increase functional ability, reduce short term mortality, and to reduce hospital readmission rates and contacts with doctors in the community for vulnerable elderly people. Medical effort is focused on those with problems amenable to medical or social intervention, and the quality of care can be audited by review of case notes or analysis of important events like hospital admission rather than by annual returns of crude process statistics that are currently required.

General practitioners are rightly critical of the contractual obligation to offer annual assessments to those aged 75 and over. A considerable minority do not honour this obligation,[6] and anecdotal evidence suggests that many fail to be systematic and comprehensive. The danger in this situation is that assessment of elderly patients may be discredited because of the imposition of an unfocussed screening programme that underemphasises the need for proper case management. General practitioners cannot abandon elderly people with significant medical problems or impairments but may be better employed in case finding, developing a database for the elderly population of the practice, auditing the quality of care, and developing teamwork skills.

The relation of disability to age suggests that the contractual obligation to assess elderly patients should be more flexible, with more home visiting of very elderly people and less of younger elderly people. The use of a two stage system with more frequent assessment at later ages may be more appropriate for elderly people and closer to the problem solving tradition of general practice than a single assessment package applied to those aged 75 and over as if they were a homogeneous population. Ideally these hypotheses should be tested in randomised controlled trials of focused interventions aimed at reducing the impact of incontinence, reducing impairment of vision and hearing, increasing functional ability, and treating depression, probably in younger age groups. In the meantime general practitioners can usefully interpret their contractual obligation to offer assessments to elderly people in creative ways, the better to develop appropriate, patient centred, and cost-effective approaches to case finding and case management.

Practice points

1 A systematic approach to functional and medical assessment of older people in the community is needed, but the 1990 contractual obligation as presently configured does not seems to meet this need. Its focus on functional ability is correct, but it needs to be more flexible in its applications in terms of the target age groups and the pattern and timing of assessments.

2 The electronic medical record can be the basis for a comprehensive profile of the health and functional ability of older people and can be fed from a number of streams:

- Opportunist brief assessments by general practitioners
- In depth assessments with standardised instruments, by doctors, nurses, social workers, and others
- Reviews from hospital specialists, professions allied to medicine (PAMS), and others.

At present electronic medical records available to general practitioners are unlikely to allow data capture with such flexibility and to the required level of complexity, but a quantum leap in practice software is imminent and development of decision support and database software specifically for these purposes is now needed.

3 The NHS has not given priority to the development of assessment programmes for older people since 1990, but this can be remedied by:

- The development of professional training programmes, especially but not exclusively designed for practice and community nurses, that will reorientate practice staff towards flexible approaches to assessment of older people
- Encouraging practices to develop a "base up" approach to meeting need among older people, with provision of appropriate resources and documentation of development in practice annual reports
- Promotion of joint working between social services, general practices, and specialists in medicine for older people at practice or locality level, perhaps using "one stop shop" models.

Practitioners should consider how best to:

- Identify those older patients who need frequent review because they have multiple problems and severe functional impairment and establish a system for such a review
- Configure their electronic medical record to collect and analyse data about the health of their older patients so that the record is usable by different professionals regardless of whether the person is able, well, and an occasional attender; or disabled, ill, and frequently seen
- Construct a package of assessment procedures that are comprehensible to the patient, possible for primary care workers to use, and comprehensive.

The package can be developed according to local need and resources from the template below. The key scales that can be used at case finding and assessment levels can be found in the Royal College of General Practitioners monograph on assessment of older people and are:

(1) The 15 item geriatric depression scale (GDS15)

119

(2) The mini-mental state examination (MMSE) or the abbreviated mental test score (AMTS) for cognitive impairment

(3) The Katz activities of daily living scale (ADL).

Geriatric depression scale

1 Are you basically satisfied with your life?   yes/NO
2 Have you dropped many of your activities and interests?   YES/no
3 Do you feel that your life is empty?   YES/no
4 Do you often get bored?   YES/no
5 Are you in good spirits most of the time?   yes/NO
6 Are you afraid that something bad is going to happen to you?   YES/no
7 Do you feel happy most of the time?   yes/NO
8 Do you often feel helpless?   YES/no
9 Do you prefer to stay at home, rather than going out and doing new things?   YES/no
10 Do you feel you have more problems with memory than most?   YES/no
11 Do you think it is wonderful to be alive now?   yes/NO
12 Do you feel pretty worthless the way you are now?   YES/no
13 Do you feel full of energy?   yes/NO
14 Do you feel that your situation is hopeless?   YES/no
15 Do you think that most people are better off than you are?   YES/no

Scoring: Answers indicating depression are in capitals. Each scores one point. Scores greater than 5 indicate probable depression.

Abbreviated mental test score

1 Age
2 Time
3 Address for recall at end of test—this should be repeated by the patient to ensure it has been heard correctly—for example, 42 West Street
4 Year

5 Name of institution
6 Recognition of two people (doctor, nurse, etc,)
7 Date of birth (day and month sufficient)
8 Year of First World War
9 Name of present monarch
10 Count backwards from 20 to 1

Scoring: Each correct answer scores one mark. A guide to rating cognitive function: 0–3 severe impairment; 4–7 moderate impairment; 8–10 normal.

Not only are these instruments not diagnostic, however, but they are likely to be of limited value in situations where the practitioner has limited contact with other local services that can provide necessary support and intervention. The key to effective assessment is knowledge of and access to other relevant services.

1 Department of Health. *A new contract for general practice.* London: HMSO, 1990.
2 Harris A. Health checks for the over-75s; the doubt persists. *BMJ* 1992;305: 599–600.
3 Freer CB. Detecting hidden needs in the elderly: screening or case finding. In: Taylor RC, Buckley EG, eds. *Preventive Care of the Elderly.* London: Royal College of General Practitioners, 1987. (Occasional paper 35).
4 RCGP. *Care of old people: a framework for progress.* London: Royal College of General Practitioners, 1990:9–10. (Occasional paper 45).
5 Philp I, ed. *Assessing elderly people in hospital and community care.* London: Farrand Press, 1994.
6 Brown K, Williams E, Groom L. Health checks on patients 75 years and over in Nottinghamshire after the new GP contract. *BMJ* 1992;305:619–21.
7 Stuck AE, Siu AL, Wieland GD, *et al.* Comprehensive geriatric assessment: a meta-analysis of controlled trials. *Lancet* 1993;342:1032–6.
8 Glendenning C, Chew C, Wilkin D. *GP assessments of patients 75 and over: the views of FHSA managers.* Manchester: Centre for Primary Care Research, University of Manchester, 1992.
9 Iliffe S, Gould MM, Wallace P. *Evaluation of the 75 and over assessments in general practice: report to the NHS Executive.* London: Department of Primary Care and Population Sciences, Royal Free Hospital Medical School, 1997.
10 Pathy MS, Bayer A, Harding K, Dibble A. Randomised trial of case finding and surveillance of elderly people at home. *Lancet* 1992;340:890–3.
11 Vetter NJ, Lewis PA, Llewellyn D. Is there a right age for case finding in elderly people? *Age Ageing* 1993;22:121–4.
12 Iliffe S, Tai S, Haines A, *et al.* Are the elderly alone an at–risk group? *BMJ* 1992;305:1001–4.

13 Iliffe S, Haines A, Stein A, *et al*. Assessment of elderly people in general practice. 3: Confiding relationships and depression. *Br J Gen Pract* 1991;41:459–61.
14 Iliffe S, Gallivan S, Haines AP, *et al*. Assessment of elderly people in general practice. 2: Functional abilities and medical problems. Br J Gen Pract 1991; 41:13–5.
15 Hickish G. Hearing problems of elderly people *BMJ* 1989;301:1415–6.
16 Gurland BJ, Cross PS. Epidemiology of psychopathology in old age: some implications for clinical services. *Psych Clin N Am* 1982;5:11–26.
17 Iliffe S, Mitchley S, Haines A. Evaluation of brief screening instruments for dementia, depression and problem drinking in general practice. *Br J Gen Pract* 1994;44:503–7.
18 MacDonald A. Do general practitioners "miss" depression in elderly patients? *BMJ* 1986;292:1365–7.
19 Pollitt B, O'Connor DW, Anderson I. Mild dementia: perception and problems. *Age Soc* 1989;9:261–75.
20 Ineichen B. Managing demented older people in the community: a review. *Family Practice* 1994;11:210–15.
21 Antonelli Incalzi R, Ineichen B, *et al*. Unrecognised dementia: sociodemographic correlates *Aging (Milano)* 1992;4:327–32.
22 Bowling A. The prevalence of psychiatric morbidity among people aged 85 and over living at home: associations with reported somatic symptoms and with consulting behaviour. *Soc Psychiatry Psychiatr Epidemiol* 1990;25:132–40.
23 O'Connor DW, Pollitt PA, Hyde JB, *et al*. Do general practitioners miss dementia in elderly patients? *BMJ* 1988;297:1107–10.
24 De Lepeleire JA, Incalzi R, *et al*. How do general practitioners diagnose dementia? *Family Practice* 1994;11:148–52.
25 MacKenzie DM. Screening the mental state of the over 75s in the community: what are GPs doing? *Psych Bull* 1992;16:146–7.
26 Hall RPG, Channing DM. Age, pattern of consultation and functional disability in elderly patients in one general practice. *BMJ* 1990;301:424–8.

6 Hospital–community interface

The likelihood of a hospital admission naturally increases with age and frailty. Elderly people are high users of hospital services; at any one time older people occupy nearly half of all hospital beds across the specialties.

A recognition that frail elderly people have special health needs—with non-specific presentation of illness, multiple pathology, altered pharmacokinetics and pharmacodynamics, and a need for a functional and social assessment and rehabilitation—has led to the development of specialist medical services for older people. The specialty of geriatric medicine in the NHS grew out of Warren's pioneering rehabilitative approach on the chronic sick wards in the 1940s. Over the past 50 years the care of older people in hospitals has been revolutionised—a national waiting list of 54 000 elderly people waiting for a hospital bed disappeared. Specialist departments providing medical care for older people have developed throughout the service, although older people are of course still admitted to other departments for specialist procedures—for example, general and orthopaedic surgery. These specialist medical services for the health care of older people may operate under various names—geriatric medicine, medicine for the elderly, care of the elderly, etc, and may have different models of care with differing admission policies.

The needs related model

Patients entering the geriatric service are selected by non-geriatricians, usually the general practitioners, who refer the patients to hospital, but selection may take place by medical staff in the accident and emergency department after an initial assessment. Particular problems such as confusional states or recurrent falls may be identified as automatically appropriate for geriatric care.

The age defined model

All medical patients above a certain age referred to hospital are admitted to the geriatric service—the age may vary from 65 to 85. The model has been justified on biological grounds, although this is not clear cut and research has not proved that age is a valid screening variable for separating those patients who would do better under geriatric than general (internal) medical care. The defining age group is usually chosen on the pragmatic grounds of the number of patients with which a geriatric service can cope within its current allocation of acute care beds.

The integrated model

Physicians with a special responsibility for the elderly service act as members of multiconsultant medical teams and take equal part in acute medical emergency work. They are also responsible for providing specialist geriatric services including rehabilitation, continuing care, day hospital, outpatients, and community liaison work.

There are argued advantages and disadvantages to all these models but no definitive answer as to which model is to be preferred. There has been no formal comparison of cost effectiveness. It is often local circumstances, constraints on resources, and staffing issues which provide the rationale for a particular style of service.[1] In 1993 geriatricians were asked to describe their styles of service: 27% operated a needs related model, 54% an age defined model, and 19% an integrated model.

Specialist services for the care of elderly people with mental health problems have also developed, usually within departments of psychiatry, although they may occasionally be integrated with the specialist medical services. These specialist services will have facilities for acute care and rehabilitation and may have some responsibility for continuing hospital care, although this role has greatly diminished in recent years. Around three quarters of admissions are unplanned—in 1990 the Audit Commission found that 37% of admissions to medical and geriatric specialties followed referral from general practitioners, a further 37% were self referrals to the accident and emergency services, and an additional 13% were urgent admissions (usually through outpatients or after a domiciliary visit).

High quality services

High quality specialist services for elderly people can be measured against criteria laid down in a number of recent documents giving advice to providers of the service and to purchasers.[1,2]

High quality health services for elderly people

- Are accessible
- Provide a spectrum of care
- Have high quality staff
- Work in a multidisciplinary way
- Are responsive to carers and users

The aim is to provide the right type of service by the right provider at the right time and place. All health services for elderly people need to be accessible, provide a spectrum of care, have good quality staff, have effective multidisciplinary working, and be responsive to carers and users.

Accessibility

Admissions should be accepted without delay, with no long waiting lists in outpatient departments. The availability of beds will depend on a good throughput of patients, which in turn depends on active rehabilitation and planning of discharge. Services should be as close to patients homes as possible to enable relatives and other carers to visit easily and to facilitate good discharge planning.

Spectrum of care—Prompt access to all diagnostic options is necessary and speedy treatment of medical problems, but a full functional and social assessment is also necessary with an active rehabilitation programme which is begun as soon as the patient's

125

condition is stabilised. Good after care is essential, either by providing ongoing medical supervision in outpatients or specific therapies in day hospital setting, or by good communication with general practitioners and other community services.

Good quality staff—Staff need to be knowledgeable about the health problems of elderly people, to be able to undertake comprehensive assessment of their needs, to be responsive to their individual circumstances, to recognise that older people themselves need to be involved in their treatment options, and to be committed to effective multidisciplinary working.

Effective multidiscplinary working—Health service staff from a number of disciplines will be involved in delivering care to an elderly person in hospital—doctors, nurses, therapists such as occupational therapists, physiotherapists, speech and language therapists, etc, as well as social workers, who may work within a hospital social work department or work in the community social services. Effective team working and communication is essential if the skills from all the disciplines are to be coordinated into effective treatment plans and effective discharge planning.

Responsive to users and carers—The individual patient will have views as to acceptability of treatment and arrangements for after discharge, and these must be taken into account. They need adequate understandable information to enable them to reach informed decisions. The particular needs of ethnic minority patients need to be met, with adequate translation services and cultural awareness. Carers and relatives also need information and to be involved in discussions about treatment options (with the permission of the patient). There may be a tension when the needs and wants of patients and carers are in conflict, and staff need to have the skills to work through these difficult situations. Patients and carers also need to know about the complaints procedure.

Rehabilitation

Rehabilitation is difficult to define. It may be thought of as a reduction of functional deficits without necessarily reversing the underlying biology of disease.[3] There will be an increase in the very elderly population over the next few decades, and the major neurological and musculoskeletal causes of disability—such as Parkinson's disease, osteoarthritis, stroke, and Alzheimer's disease—increase almost exponentially with age so there is a reasonable assumption that the need for rehabilitation of elderly people will increase.

Classification of the differences between impairment, disability, and handicap has helped to clarify the concept of rehabilitation.[4]

- **Impairment** is any loss or abnormality of psychological, physiological, or anatomical structure or function.
- **Disability** is the restriction or lack of ability to perform a task or activity—for example, walking, dressing.
- **Handicap** is the resultant social disadvantage and dependency—for example, reading a newspaper, going to the shops, gardening.

The amount of handicap need not be proportional to the amount of impairment—a person may have only a small impairment and yet be enormously handicapped or be severely impaired and yet be relatively free of handicap.

Doctors tend to be most familiar with uncovering illnesses and impairments (the diagnosis), but patients with chronic disease are often more concerned with the consequences of their disease (disability and handicap).

Rehabilitation is mainly about intervening between impairment and disabilities and disabilities and handicaps. A person suffering from a disease is not simply a biological organism but an individual in a complex environment. Rehabilitation therefore has to take place at several levels.

Social and psychological areas need to be dealt with as well as physical function. General encouragement, advice, education, and listening to patients are essential, as well as specific treatment programmes to try and optimise function.[5]

A thorough assessment is necessary and may include an evaluation of disability with the Barthel index.[6,7] When used at repeated intervals, this index can be used to measure the progress of rehabilitation. The main disadvantage is that it can be insensitive to change and it has a low "ceiling"—patients may achieve a high score but still be unable to go out, cook, etc.

Barthel index

Bowels

0	Incontinent (or needs to be given enema)
1	Occasional accident (once a week)
2	Continent

Bladder

0	Incontinent or catheterised and unable to manage alone
1	Occasional accident (maximum once per 24 hours)
2	Continent (for more than seven days)

Grooming

0	Needs help with personal care: face, hair, teeth, shaving
1	Independent (implements provided)

Toilet use

0	Dependent
1	Needs some help but can do something alone
2	Independent (on and off, wiping, dressing)

Feeding

0	Unable
1	Needs help in cutting, spreading butter, etc.
2	Independent

Transfer

0	Unable—no sitting balance
1	Major help (physical, one or two people); can sit
2	Minor help (verbal or physical)
3	Independent

Mobility

0	Immobile
1	Wheelchair independent, including corners, etc.
2	Walks with help (verbal or physical) of one person
3	Independent (but may use an aid)

Dressing

0	Dependent
1	Needs help but can do about half unaided
2	Independent (including buttons, zips, laces, etc)

Barthel index—*continued*

Stairs

0	Unable
1	Needs help (verbal, physical, carrying aid)
2	Independent up and down

Bathing

0	Dependent
1	Independent (or in shower)

NOTE: Measure what the patient does, not what they *can* do.

Specific goals should be set in consultation with the patient, care giver, and members of the rehabilitation team. The goals should be explicit, documented, and achievable and have a clear time frame when the situation will be reassessed. Various disciplines will be involved, and good multidisciplinary working is essential. Physiotherapists, nurses, occupational therapists, speech therapists, dieticians, medical staff, social workers, and community liaison staff are some of the specialists who may be involved in the assessment and carrying out of an agreed treatment plan.

Sometimes patients do not make the expected progress. Common reasons are undiagnosed medical problems including adverse reactions to medication, occult depression or dementia, communications difficulties, and underlying psychological problems affecting motivation.

Research showing the success of individual treatments is sparse, although there is evidence that physiotherapy has improved functioning in stroke[8,9] and that the overall impact on the patient of a rehabilitation package improves activities of daily living scores.[10] There is evidence that liaison between orthopaedic and geriatric units for the rehabilitation of elderly people with fractured neck of femur gives improved outcomes for patients, and stroke units have been shown to be effective. Provision of aids—for example, to help with mobility or with cooking—can also enhance independence, and aids are becoming more sophisticated and better tailored to individual needs.

129

Effective team working is essential among the different disciplines, and this is one of the major challenges to professional staff working in rehabilitation. Joint training initiatives can be helpful, and regular case conferences should be held. The use of collaborative care planning and one set of notes for all disciplines also helps effective interdisciplinary working.

Rehabilitation needs to begin as early as possible after an acute event—for example, stroke, fractured neck of femur—although some patients with a chronic disability such as arthritis may also need rehabilitation if their functioning has slowly deteriorated.

Rehabilitation can take place in various settings—on an acute hospital ward, in a specialised rehabilitation ward or highly specialised unit such as for stroke, or in the community. The choice of the settings will depend on the presentation of the patient, their dependency and care needs, especially at night, and the complexity of the disability. Much rehabilitation will be started in a hospital acute ward after an acute episode such as stroke and will be continued in a specialised rehabilitation area and then continued in the community.

Circumstances of poor housing and social support and lack of domiciliary rehabilitation services may mean it is more appropriate to continue rehabilitation as an inpatient rather than at home. Low dependency and less complex disability in a setting of appropriate housing and domestic circumstances may mean rehabilitation can be delivered at home. Community occupational therapists and physiotherapists can do assessments at home and develop a goal orientated treatment plan which can be supervised by professionals, by carers, or carried through by the patient themselves (see chapter 4). Coordination and team working is more difficult in the community, and various different agencies may be involved in, for example, the provision of aids and adaptations. This is one of the challenges for professionals in the community. To develop good interdisciplinary working relationships a key worker needs to coordinate the treatment plan—this may be a therapist, nurse, or the general practitioner. Stroke rehabilitation at home has been evaluated,[11] and interventions with patients with rheumatoid arthritis, Parkinson's disease, and falls have been shown to be effective. Provision of aids has been shown to promote independence.

Hospital at Home schemes may provide ongoing rehabilitation with special community rehabilitation teams. Patients can also

Case study: Mr T

Mr T, 92, was admitted to hospital after a fall. He was found lying on the floor in the bathroom of his terraced house after 8 hours by a neighbour who has a key. Medical examination showed he was in rapid atrial fibrillation, and he was given digoxin; there was no definite evidence of a myocardial infarction. Investigations revealed no other medical process. He was referred to physiotherapy and occupational therapy. He had poor mobility and had lost his confidence. He was able to dress himself slowly. He was transferred to the rehabilitation ward for further physiotherapy and dressing practice. The multidisciplinary team discussed his discharge at the weekly case conference. He had difficulty in climbing stairs, and it was suggested that the bed be brought downstairs. His son was able to arrange this. He was able to move around with a Zimmer frame and would need a chemical toilet downstairs, arranged by the occupational therapist. He was able to prepare simple meals but took a long time. Meals on Wheels were offered two days a week through social services, and his son agreed to take in a hot meal at the weekend. His neighbour normally did the shopping for him. He had never applied for the attendance allowance, and the social worker agreed to help him with the forms. A pendant alarm was arranged through social services. A home visit was made by the occupational therapist and occupational therapy aide, who found loose rugs and a difficult step between the living room and kitchen. His son was asked to remove the rugs and to put a handrail near the step.

Mr T was discharged home after 23 days, with a follow up outpatient appointment to monitor his atrial fibrillation. His general practitioner was sent a discharge summary documenting the diagnosis, medication, functional ability, and support services offered at discharge.

attend outpatient services for specialist rehabilitation—for example, infrared therapy, hydrotherapy, etc. They can also attend a geriatric day hospital to receive specific treatments to enable them to work towards a specific goal. This will usually be for a defined period, two to three months usually, with regular review and evaluation of the treatment against the goals. While all day hospital care will provide some social stimulation and support, the main aim is to be part of a rehabilitation programme. Once a patient has reached the optimum goal or a further assessment has indicated that a new goal has to be defined, which may not necessitate ongoing treatment, the patient will be discharged. If patients need further social support other facilities need to be explored, such as local authority or voluntary day centres, day care in the private sector, or luncheon clubs, etc.

As discussed above, many older people in hospital are not within a specialised service for elderly people. There have been widespread improvements in access to acute care for older people, but there are still difficulties in after acute care. Sometimes the term rehabilitation can conjure up images of highly specialised services for patients with a very complex disability, and there has been a misunderstanding that rehabilitation can be done only in very specialised settings. All elderly people need assessment of their function and holistic goal orientated team care before being discharged from hospital, however, and the term "post acute care" has been developed to mean a more generic form of rehabilitation that encompasses the principles of specialist care of older people. Post acute care should be available to all older people who need it irrespective of type of hospital, ward, and speciality. Poor quality post acute care has recently been documented by the Audit Commission report on services for people with fractured neck of femur[12] and in reports by the health service commissioner.

Elderly people with fractured neck of femur need a full medical assessment to establish the reasons why they fell and to diagnose and treat concomitant medical problems. They also need rehabilitation to begin immediately they have recovered from surgery and adequate nutrition, attention to pressure areas, promotion of continence, and management of pain. The Audit Commission found varying degrees of compliance with these standards in a survey of nine hospitals. Varying arrangements for ongoing rehabilitation were in place, from rehabilitation taking place on the orthopaedic ward with referral to specialist services for elderly people only if a patient was seen to be "blocking" an orthopaedic bed to a more structured liaison with elderly care physicians. They may regularly visit orthopaedic wards to give advice and the patients are then promptly transferred to a specialist rehabilitation ward if rehabilitation is to take a long time, or arrangements may be in place for the elderly care physician to see all patients admitted before the operation and to advise on subsequent management and rehabilitation. Precise arrangements will vary from hospital to hospital, but it is recommended that clear protocols are in place so everyone is clear when referrals should be made and what facilities for post acute care and rehabilitation are in place.

The emphasis on a fast turnover of patients by trusts may lead to inappropriate early discharge to private nursing homes (a comparison with the "warehousing" of the past in long stay geriatric wards).

There are persistent attitudinal problems in NHS staff towards older people, who can be seen as "blocking beds" on acute medical wards or after surgery; these attitudes are the result of poor training, understaffing, and failures in the system.

The principles of rehabilitation, with a thorough assessment taking into account the views of the patients and the carers, a goal orientated care plan, good multidisciplinary working, and effective discharge planning need to be applied to all post acute care of elderly people. The involvement of specialist services will vary depending on local need, for example, orthopaedic-geriatric liaison, but it is one of the challenges to the NHS at present to ensure that *all* elderly people in hospital receive appropriate assessment and rehabilitation, regardless of where they are. The Royal College of Physicians of London is due to publish guidelines on post acute care of older people in hospital for the use of purchasers and providers. Improved training in the needs of older people and the importance of rehabilitation will help to improve the situation.

Discharge planning

The interface between hospital and community is at its most critical at the time of discharge of an elderly person from hospital. Research has highlighted many difficulties in the past, and new guidelines have emerged to help overcome these difficulties.

An older person is more likely to use community services after their discharge—an increase in contacts with social workers, home helps, district nurses, and general practitioners has been documented. In the 1980s just over a third of all admissions to local authority residential care came from hospitals. These increased referrals to community services, however, should not suggest that hospitals have been uniformly successful in meeting elderly people's needs at discharge.

Patients may face difficulties if discharges have not been adequately planned, as has been shown in the literature:[13]

- A lack of preparation for discharge[14]: many elderly patients were told of their discharge only the day before or on the day itself (up to 39%)
- Little opportunity to discuss with hospital staff the difficulties patients perceive on their discharge[14]
- Lack of advice on discharge[14]: only a minority received advice on how to look after themselves and advice was often non-specific
- Lack of care on discharge[15]: some patients did not have adequate services arranged
- A risk of premature discharge[16]: a small proportion of patients thought they had been discharged too soon.

Reduce readmissions by

- Effective preparation for discharge
- Proper timing of discharge
- Adequate information to general practitioners
- Considering needs of carer
- Organising prompt nursing and social support
- General practitioner follow up
- Attention to medication

Readmission rates have been studied to see if inadequate discharge arrangements are a contributing factor. Although the most common reason for readmission to hospital is a relapse of the original medical condition, it has been shown that readmission in up to 60% of cases could have been avoided if more effective action had been taken in the following areas—preparation for and timing of discharges, attention to the needs of the carer, timely and adequate information to the general practitioner, subsequent action by the general practitioner, sufficient and prompt nursing, and social support and management of medication.[17]

Recent guidance has been issued to the NHS and social services to make discharge procedures more effective.[18,19] The various agencies involved must acknowledge their complementary responsibilities. The 1990 NHS and Community Care Act means that hospital discharge policies and procedures must also take into full account the new requirements for local authorities to undertake needs-based assessment for community care, and there is a requirement to have a jointly agreed hospital discharge procedure.

The development of systematic arrangements for the discharge of patients from hospital is of central importance both from the perspective of managerial efficiency and from concern for individual patient welfare.[20] Without such procedures in place patients may remain in hospital longer than necessary, with associated problems of bed blocking and shortage of beds for acute admissions. Conversely, patients may be discharged to inadequate and poorly organised support with the risk of deterioration and subsequent readmission.

Difficulties with timely discharge are likely to arise because of inadequacies in two areas: management of hospital resources and communication procedures. Better planning of inpatient investigations, review of patients' progress by senior medical staff who can take decisions about discharge, better organisation of transport, and take home medications could all lead to a more efficient use of medical beds. Good communication is essential, both with the individual patient and carer and also with the various professionals from different agencies in the hospital and community.

The Patient's Charter includes the discharge of patients from hospital as one of its national charter standards. It states that,

> *The charter standard is that before you are discharged from hospital a decision should be made about any continuing health or social care needs you may have. Your hospital will agree arrangements for meeting these needs with community nursing services and local authority social services departments before you are discharged. You and, with your agreement, your carers will be consulted and informed at all stages.*

A *Hospital Discharge Workbook* was published in 1994 by the NHS Executive to give detailed guidance on discharge procedures.[21]

Discharge planning can be started *before* admission if the admission is for an elective procedure. An assessment before admission will need to look at social support, the patient's functional

Hospital discharge check list

- Has appropriate transport been organised?
- Is there someone to accompany the patient if necessary and to settle them at home?
- Has full information been given to the patient about medication, dressings, and follow up arrangements?
- Have any necessary aids or adaptations been supplied?
- Have steps been taken to reactivate home care, meals on wheels, etc, on the appropriate date?
- If the patient lives alone have arrangements been made to make their home ready for their return?

ability, and predicted functional ability after the procedure—plans for aftercare can then be made.

After a patient is admitted discharge planning should begin immediately. An estimated date of discharge can be given and worked towards, which can be revised if the patient's condition deteriorates. Full information must be obtained about the patient's social circumstances, either from the patient or from various other sources—for example, relatives, carers, neighbours, warden, general practitioner, etc. A history of the patient's previous functional ability is needed in the activities of daily living—washing, dressing, mobility, toileting and continence, cooking, shopping, domestic work, etc, and what help was being given before.

The functional abilities of the patient in hospital need to be assessed; this can be a simple assessment or may need a full multidisciplinary assessment if there are complex functional problems. An individual care plan must be drawn up and, if a rehabilitation programme is being instituted, time specific goals should be set.

The views of older people themselves and their families and carers must be taken into account. Prompt referral to other agencies, for example, social work, is essential if statutory services are to be mobilised. (There is evidence that this is done more quickly if social workers are permanently attached to the hospital in a hospital social work department than if referrals go out to the community social services.[22]) A district nurse liaison post can be very useful, working with the nurses on the ward to complete a nursing assessment which can be used in the community by district nurses and health visitors and to predict what nursing services will be needed.

Specialist nursing skills, such as in psychiatric nursing or continence advice, may be used as part of the assessment.

If the needs of a patient are complex and there will be complex ongoing support in the community with many different agencies, both private and public sector, and a need for coordination of such a care package, a full multidisciplinary case conference can be called and a care management plan drawn up to be implemented on discharge. A key worker in the community, the care manager, will be nominated to have ongoing responsibility for ensuring that the support is sufficient and appropriate—this is usually a social worker but need not necessarily be so, it could be a district nurse, occupational therapist, etc.

Sometimes a home visit will be undertaken to assess the home circumstances. Adaptations may be needed—for example, banisters, grab rails, ramps—or furniture may need to be rearranged—for example, loose rugs removed, bed brought downstairs. The patient's abilities may be much better in familiar home circumstances, cooking a meal in a familiar kitchen, for example, or the visit may highlight new problems which will need a solution. Home visits are usually done by occupational therapists, who may go with another professional such as a social worker or physiotherapist. Care givers and family members should usually be invited to attend the home assessment visit.

Good communication between all the agencies is essential, and the discharge plan must be documented and shared with the patient. The patient needs information about what services and aftercare are being provided, as well as information about their condition and prognosis. A full explanation about medication is essential—non-compliance with medication regimens may be nearly 50%,[23] and the patient needs to understand any new medications, what to do with tablets they may have at home, for how long medications are to be taken, what to do when the tablets run out, and any potential side effects.

Team working skills are needed and should be fostered; interprofessional rivalries and differences of culture within organisations need to be understood and worked through, training may help. For example, a hospital may run a series of small workshops to which nursing staff, therapy staff, and medical staff are invited, to work through issues around discharge of patients; a problem solving approach is useful.

The outcome of the assessment for discharge may be an opinion reached by the multidisciplinary team that the patient would be at risk if they returned to their home circumstances, even with added community support, and continuing care in some sort of residential or nursing home is needed. This opinion must obviously be shared by the patient and reached only after a full multidisciplinary assessment and attempt at rehabilitation have been completed. Decisions will then be made with the patient, family members, and care givers as to an appropriate and acceptable placement. Sometimes an elderly person will not accept the advice of the multidisciplinary team that they are not safe to be at home and will insist on returning there. Unless they are shown to be completely incapable of making a decision, which would involve an assessment by a consultant psychiatrist and a section under the Mental Health Act (which is very rarely applied in these circumstances), the elderly person has a right to live at home "at risk". Services should be put in place to support the elderly person. A patient cannot be forced to go to a residential or nursing home against his or her will. The decision to return home may cause distress in family members, who may feel worried about their safety and unduly burdened by the demands the elderly person will make on them at home. The lack of coercive powers needs to be explained carefully and sensitively to care givers, and the situation will need to be kept under review in the community.

At the time of discharge, arrangements should be communicated with the patient and carers and to the community staff who will be involved in ongoing support. Communication with the general practitioner is essential; this may be done by telephone or by a short discharge summary which is sent at the time of discharge (a fuller summary may follow). Development of information technology has improved this communication—for example, fax, and email, though procedures to preserve confidentiality of patient data must be strictly followed.

The community based health and social service practitioners then need to react in a timely and appropriate way to give the ongoing support needed after discharge. Further assessments may

Case Study: Mrs S

Mrs S, 84, has lived alone since she was widowed 10 years ago. Her daughters call in, but she has refused other help. She has become more vague over the past two years and was admitted to hospital with a chest infection and acute confusional state. She made a good recovery, but her mental state was found to be impaired (mental test score 5/10). She is mobile and continent but has some difficulties dressing herself. She is adamant she wants to go home. Her daughters express great concern about her living alone again and feel they will have to resume responsibility for her wellbeing. She has been ringing them up several times a day and sometimes at night. She is known to the local social services but has refused Meals on Wheels and home care. The daughters thought she should be in residential care. The consultant and hospital social worker explain to the family that she cannot be discharged to a residential home against her will. She is still competent to make decisions even though she is unrealistic about her abilities. The consultant agrees to get a psychiatric opinion—the old age psychiatrist agrees that she cannot be deemed incompetent. Discharge arrangements are therefore made—a home visit is done, and she is thought to be "at risk" if she does not accept home care in the mornings to help her wash and dress and Meals on Wheels. These services are arranged and her case is passed to a community social worker who will organise the package of care. The family are worried but are given the name of the community social worker. Her general practitioner is informed by phone of the discharge arrangements.

Mrs S is discharged home 14 days after her admission, but shortly after her discharge refuses to allow the home care worker and Meals on Wheels to come in.

be made in the community if needs change and a new care plan may be implemented.

Explicit procedures and protocols are essential for good discharge arrangements, so everyone knows exactly who is responsible for what and when. Explicit aftercare arrangements are also needed—is there to be an outpatient follow up, is the general practitioner to visit, are there attendances at the day hospital or day centre, etc, —and the patient needs to know who to contact in the case of difficulty. The person the patient chooses to contact will often be the general practitioner, who will therefore be put in the role of the key worker for the patient. It is essential that the general practitioner is fully aware of all the discharge arrangements and knows who to contact if there are problems. Sometimes, there are arrangements for *all* elderly people discharged from hospital to receive a follow up visit by a district nurse or health visitor within 72 hours, although selective visits may be a better use of resources.

There may be particular difficulties with discharges for patients who decide to discharge themselves as arrangements may not be in place or for people who are unwilling to be discharged or whose family or carers do not want them discharged. These situations need to be sensitively handled and need a lot of counselling and communication skills. Discharges of frail elderly people who live alone should not usually take place on Friday afternoons or at weekends and bank holidays if the statutory services are not available.

Pointers to difficulties with discharge

- Unplanned admission
- Living alone
- No regular visitors in hospital
- Mental impairment

Another area of particular difficulty is elderly people who present to the accident and emergency facility and who are not admitted. Explicit procedures for follow up of these patients is needed; some accident and emergency departments have liaison staff who then notify the community services and the general practitioner so that a follow up visit can take place within 24 hours.

Care needs to be taken with patients who have particular communication needs to ensure they understand the discharge arrangements and have contributed their views—for example, those from ethnic minorities and those with learning disabilities, speech and language problems, or hearing difficulties.

One of the intentions of the new arrangements for community care and the introduction of the Patient's Charter was to improve arrangements for hospital discharge, particularly of frail elderly people. It is a requirement of the legislation that social services departments and health authorities have jointly agreed procedures in place for hospital discharges. Failures in the system were documented in 1992.[24]

Has there been any improvement? There was concern when the changes were implemented in 1993 that there may be delay in hospital discharges because of the necessity for a full assessment of need by a social worker and lack of funding in the community for domiciliary social services or placement in residential and nursing homes. Delays in assessment by a social worker, particularly if he or she is based in the local authority and not as part of a hospital social work team or if the patient lives in a different local authority to the one in which the hospital is situated, can lead to an increased length of stay.[25] Some hospitals have found difficulty in discharging elderly people to residential and nursing homes because of a lack of local authority funding because of cash limits, and this has led to "bed blocking". Patients also need time to make a choice of a suitable placement, particularly if they are to move to a nursing or residential home. There are also continued delays in supplying aids and adaptations. Despite these difficulties, however, some studies have shown that discharge arrangements are working better, and there has been a reduction in hospital length of stay,[26] although other early studies did not confirm this.[27]

Discharges from hospital to residential or nursing home care have been evaluated[28,29]: wide variations in practice were found. The level of social services activity in hospitals had increased and many organisations had made a lot of effort to facilitate interagency working and speedy responses, with few cases needing to go to dispute procedures. Difficulties were encountered with the widely differing provision in the NHS for ongoing rehabilitation, however, with increased emphasis on early discharge to free up beds for acute admissions. As a consequence patients were not given time to realise their full potential for recovery, confusion arose about access to continuing health care provision, and there was little separate assessment of carers' needs. There were also difficulties with patients exercising choice about their placement in a particular nursing or residential home because of the pressure for them to leave hospital quickly. Recommendations have been made jointly by the NHS Executive and Social Services Inspectorate that there should be convalescence or recovery time to prevent entry into long stay care. Management systems and multidisciplinary training should be improved so that assessment and discharge procedures can improve, assessments in hospital should be more "outward looking", involving staff based in the community, there should be a choice of home—and older people may need extra time and support to exercise that choice, and that there should be substantial improvements in planning of care.

The Audit Commission report on the coordination of care for elderly people with hip fractures also documented poor discharge planning and a need for early identification of needs, adequate rehabilitation, and a full assessment and planning of support needed.[12] Few hospitals had adequate procedures in place. There was little awareness by ward staff of discharge policies, and multidisciplinary meetings were not held regularly. Poor monitoring of discharges and readmissions was usual, and training staff in assessment procedures was often inadequate.

The appointment of discharge liaison nurses may have hindered the involvement of ward staff who then abdicated responsibility, and it is important that liaison nurses facilitate the ward staff to implement good discharges. Joint training would be helpful. The ability of organisations to deliver good practice is still inadequate, and much more work needs to be done, both organisationally and in delivering adequate training to staff.

The role of specialist services

Hospital services

The development of specialist geriatric services grew out of the application of principles of rehabilitation to elderly chronically sick patients in the wards of institutions after the second world war. The abdication of responsibility of the specialist medical services towards elderly people because of an assumption that disability and infirmity were the result of old age itself and not ill health left a vacuum which was filled by the pioneers of what was to become the speciality of geriatric medicine. Gradually, hospital services devoted to the care of elderly people were established in the NHS. The emphasis moved from continuing care of old people in what were often the old workhouse buildings to active diagnosis and treatment of illness in elderly people and rehabilitation of functional disability. The knowledge base of illness in old age and the aging process itself increased with the application of research methods and establishment of academic departments. The specialty has fostered attitudes of holistic care, accurate early diagnosis and treatment, early rehabilitation, multidisciplinary working, and good interagency working.[30]

It can be argued, however, that to separate out the care of elderly people to services defined by age is itself discriminatory. There is a danger of deprivation of access to other specialist medical services and putting the medical care of elderly people in a ghetto. Ageism exists in our society and therefore specialist services for older people may in their own way stigmatise them. Age itself may not be a discriminator for disability—there are no clear chronological markers and the elderly population is heterogeneous not homogeneous.

The future of specialist hospital services for older people is therefore under debate. Some argue that the way forward is to incorporate the knowledge of geriatric medicine into the whole spectrum of medical practice and to abandon the specialty altogether; this assumes that ageism does not exist, however, and that older people will not be discriminated against in terms of access and treatment within medical practice, and there are still strong arguments for maintaining specialist services which will focus on the needs of those individuals. It is true now that elderly people sometimes have to wait longer for investigations, such as barium enemas for radiology, because of the mistaken belief that they will not benefit from treatment. Within the internal market, health authorities and general practitioner fund holders are looking to providers to give the most value for money and there are incentives within the system not to refer elderly people for treatment. Provider units need to maximise finished consultant episodes to maintain the efficiency index, so there are incentives to reduce length of stay and to discharge early to the community. These tensions are leading to widespread debate about the future shape of services. Some trusts have abdicated involvement in specialist inpatient rehabilitation and placed such services in the community in a domiciliary setting. Separate hospital and community trusts have also contributed to increased difficulties of working aims and different bureaucratic structures; the separation of social services into purchaser and provider arms has also increased difficulties working across the interfaces.

There has also been encouragement for older people to buy commercial medical care with tax relief on private health insurance.

Many plans exclude access to treatment of chronic disease, rehabilitation and continuing care, however, and therefore the "benefits" are irrelevant to the needs of many older people.

Possible future roles for specialist medical staff working in geriatric medicine can be postulated; the future may see a combination of these roles or the service may develop in one particular direction. Specialist geriatricians may continue to be hospital based clinical and research physicians as now. The process of integration with general medicine may continue so that geriatricians do a full range of all age acute medical care but maintain responsibility for rehabilitation and consultation for older people. Some geriatricians may develop their role as epidemiologists and advocates for services for older people and become advisers to purchasers.

Community services

Some consultant geriatricians have worked more in the community than in hospital and the role of the community geriatrician may develop in future, although there are only a few posts nationally at present.[31] This has sometimes been taken to mean specialist geriatric medicine as practised in rural areas. Rural areas are likely to have more facilities spread throughout the district outside the district general hospital, but most secondary care still takes place within hospital settings—for example, community hospitals. The organisation of services providing medical care for older people at home, however, is as appropriate in urban as well as rural areas. The word "community" can refer to any activity outside the district general hospital at one extreme to seeing patients either at home or in primary care settings. Medical services for older people are seen by some as a possible area where traditional secondary care could be provided outside hospitals. If this were the case frail elderly people would still need to access the specialist knowledge a consultant geriatrician has and therefore the post of community geriatrician has been mooted. It is thought, however, that even if the emphasis is on work outside the hospital a specialist physician should be part of a department of geriatric medicine and have some responsibility for inpatient care, otherwise the post would be isolated and unsupported.[32]

Specialist work in the community can include assessment for residential care, responsibility for elderly people in community

144

hospitals, and care at home schemes for those who are severely disabled.

There is an increasing need for advice and support to general practitioners as they become responsible for more severely dependent older people both in residential care and in their own home but especially in nursing homes. New avenues of community involvement could include clinics in health centres and the establishment of local community teams with nursing and social services staff leading to the identification of at risk patients. Liaison with social services, private and voluntary sector, contribution to planning services, and setting assessment criteria are roles which can also be developed. Specialists in the mental health of older people—old age psychiatrists—also have a major role in the community, they often assess people in their own homes and have a large role in liaison with primary care.

The white paper *Caring for People* and the subsequent National Health Service Community Care Act gave social services departments of local authorities the responsibility for assessing the needs of older people and arranging for care in their own home or in residential care. The assessment should include medical advice as to the possibility of medical intervention lessening the need for care. Accurate diagnosis, treatment, and rehabilitation may reduce dependency and disability and the need for supportive services. The legislation does not make it clear whether medical advice should include a specialist opinion rather than be given by the patients' own general practitioner; this has been an area of contention within the medical profession.

There is agreement that while a patient remains in hospital and under the clinical responsibility of the consultant it is appropriate that a hospital specialist (who may not be the same specialist that the patient has caring for them on their initial admission to hospital) should perform the relevant medical assessment at the request of social services. The relevant assessment details and recommendations should be communicated to the general practitioner. If a general practitioner is a fund holder who has become responsible for purchasing community care, it is imperative that they are knowingly involved at an early stage in the assessment process so that any implications of community staff time and associated cost can be dealt with and budgeted for.

The more difficult area is when a patient needs a medical assessment for care needs when she or he is at home in the community. For simple care needs, the general practitioner will provide the initial medical component of the assessment. They will have relevant medical and social data on an individual patient to assist at this stage of the assessment and can provide future recommendations for either continuing care in the community with support or alternative placement in either nursing or residential home care. It has been strongly argued, however, that no elderly person should relocate from home to a residential or nursing home, a major life event, without the benefit of a *specialist* medical opinion to see if the move could be averted by attending to reversible medical causes of disability and dependence. The general practitioner is of course able to refer the patient for a specialist opinion, either to an outpatient department or by asking for a domiciliary consultation by a consultant, but this is not mandatory—it is at the general practitioner's discretion, at present. Placement in residential or nursing home is such a major relocation that it can be argued that everything possible should be done to assure that this is the best option and that complex care needs cannot be met in any other way. If the role of medical assessment is to remain with general practitioners it is essential that they have the appropriate knowledge base and skills to undertake such an assessment, so that all appropriate interventions can be made.

This has major implications for training and ongoing education of general practitioners. Vocational training schemes for doctors planning to enter general practice need to cover principles of assessment of frail elderly people, and ongoing continuing medical education should cover this topic.

There is dissent in the profession about this matter—specialist physicians and psychiatrists dealing with old people think that there should be a requirement for a specialist opinion before placement in residential or nursing home care—general practitioners think they are well able to undertake the required medical assessment. At present, there is local variation as to how the assessments are done and by whom. In some areas, clinical medical officers may do the medical assessments for social services, though again there is a need for such doctors to be appropriately trained in the mental and physical problems which occur in old age.

If these educational needs are not met then elderly people will continue to be placed in inappropriate settings. In the future, specialist medical opinions may need to be made mandatory.

Continuing health care

The NHS was responsible for the care of the chronic sick, often elderly and frail people; long stay geriatric beds were a feature of the hospital service, often housed in old institutions—these were taken into the health service in 1948. The more active approach to treatment and rehabilitation increased the throughput in these beds, and the number of long stay patients in geriatric and psychiatry services reduced. Continuing nursing care could also be provided in the home. Often informal care was provided by families who maybe were awaiting a placement in a long stay geriatric bed; waiting lists for beds were common. A small number of people could afford placement in a private nursing home. Local authorities provided residential accommodation for elderly people, and there was a small private sector providing residential care for elderly people who could afford to pay for themselves. In the 1980s, as has already been discussed, the change in social security rules meant that many older people could access sufficient income to pay for care in private residential and nursing homes. The private sector has therefore grown enormously at the same time as a reduction in public sector continuing care beds provided in NHS hospitals and a reduction in local authority residential places have taken place.[34]

Table 6.1   Provision of long term care

Places	1983	1994
Total	280 000	465 000
NHS	55 600 (20%)	37 500 (8%)
Private/voluntary nursing homes	18 200 (6.5%)	148 500 (32%)
Local authority residential homes	115 900 (41.5%)	68 900 (15%)
Voluntary residential homes	37 600 (13%)	45 500 (10%)
Private residential homes	51 800 (19%)	164 200 (35%)

The community care legislation introduced in 1990 and implemented in 1993 aimed to control the placement of people in nursing homes by making assessment essential if they were to receive public funds. Despite this, the private sector provision for nursing and residential care has continued to grow as one of the other objectives of the legislation was to encourage further development of residential provision in the private and voluntary sector with a reduction of direct provision by local authorities. Changes in the health service with the introduction of hospital trusts have also meant a reduction in continuing care beds with an increased placement in private nursing homes. These are sometimes contracted for by the health authority, but often the individual person is assessed under the community care process, and social services pay for the bed or the individual or family is liable for the cost.

Case Study: Mrs M

Mrs M, 82, has been diagnosed with an inoperable glioma after referral to the neurosurgeons. She presented with a progressive hemiplegia and speech difficulty. She was transferred to the local community hospital under the care of the geriatrician. Her nephew insists she should stay in hospital and refuses to look for a nursing home (she owns her own house and would have to find the costs herself). She does not fit the locally agreed criteria for continuing health costs, however, although she is immobile and has language difficulty, she is alert and feeds herself. A nursing assessment has not revealed any specialist nursing requirements. She has a brain tumour but this seems to be slow growing, and she is not likely to die in the very near future, which has been locally defined as within two weeks. The consultant therefore wishes to discharge her. Her nephew insists on an appeal to a review panel, which is convened within two weeks. The independent assessor find that the criteria for continuing health care have been applied correctly and that she should not occupy an NHS bed. Her nephew is very angry that she will have to pay for nursing home costs and refuses to look for one. The hospital therefore has to find an independent advocate for Mrs M to act on her behalf to help with the discharge.

Access to local authority payments is of course means tested—the value of an older person's assets, including their home if they are owner-occupiers, is taken into account. The amount of assets which can be kept has recently been increased from £8000 to £16 000, but many elderly people have had to sell their houses and use their savings to pay for institutional care in the private sector. If a spouse is still living in the house the sale can be deferred; this does not apply if another carer is living there, such as daughter or son, who may have to move out of their parents' home to make the assets available. This is obviously impacting on the inheritance which can be passed on to the next generation.

It has given rise to the anomaly that while long term nursing care provided within a hospital is free under the NHS, long term nursing care provided in the private sector has to be paid for, either by the individual's assets or picked up through local authority funding.

There has been much debate about whether the care of these patients is the responsibility of the NHS or social services departments. Many studies have shown that residents in residential homes may have the same dependency as those in nursing homes and long stay wards in hospitals. It has not been clear which patients are entitled to free continuing health care provided by the NHS and which patients will receive means tested care, organised through social services.

It is possible for the NHS to pay for beds in private nursing homes if it is thought that the patient is still entitled to continuing health care, and thus a further anomaly is possible—that two individuals may be in the same nursing home, with the same level of disability, one who is receiving free care because they have been placed through a health service route and the other paying for the care from their own assets as they have been placed through a community care assessment by social workers or because they have chosen themselves to enter care without an assessment.

Guidance was issued in 1995 to try to clarify the situation and to confirm the responsibilities of the NHS.[33] It made clear that all health authorities (and general practitioner fund holders where applicable) must arrange and fund services including:

- Specialist medical and nursing assessment
- Rehabilitation and recovery
- Palliative health care
- Continuing inpatient care under specialist supervision in hospital or in a nursing home
- Respite health care

- Specialist health care support to people in nursing homes, residential care homes or the community.

Health authorities were required by April 1996 to have developed local policies and eligibility criteria which set out clearly the criteria to be used as the basis in individual cases for decisions about the need for NHS funded care. The range, type, location, and level of services which would be arranged and funded by the NHS to meet continuing health care needs in a particular area also had to be made explicit. These policies must be agreed by the local authority and have been subject to a period of public consultation. Thus the criteria for eligibility is locally determined and may differ from one geographical area to another. The guidance makes it clear that the decision to discharge from hospital rests with the consultant in charge, who should take into account a multidisciplinary assessment of the patient's needs and recommends that a specialist with responsibility for continuing care (including geriatricians and old age psychiatrists) should be involved if the possibility of continuing NHS inpatient care, nursing home, or residential care or an intensive package of support at home may be needed.

The guidance suggests that continuing inpatient care arranged and funded by the NHS may be indicated if the patient,

- Needs ongoing and regular specialist clinical supervision (weekly or more often) on account of the complexity, nature, or intensity of his or her medical, nursing, or other needs
- Has the need for frequent not easily predictable intervention
- Is likely to die in the very near future
- The patient needs a period of rehabilitation and recovery.

Local criteria will have been drawn up with this guidance. Some areas have very prescriptive definitions, with specific measurements of function such as the Barthel index, others have broader definitions which can be interpreted by the multidisciplinary team.

Patients and their families are entitled to information, usually in written form, about what will happen if patients need continuing care and details of what, if any, continuing care will be arranged and funded by the NHS. When patients have been assessed as not requiring NHS continuing inpatient care they do not have the right to occupy an NHS bed indefinitely. They do, however, have a right

150

to refuse to be discharged from NHS care to a nursing home or residential care home. In such cases, the social services department should work with the hospital and community based staff to explore all options. If all other options have been rejected it may be necessary for the hospital in consultation with other agencies to implement discharge to the patient's home with a package of health and social care within the options and resources available.

A patient and his or her family or carer each has the right to appeal to the health authority against a decision not to give NHS inpatient continuing care. A response should be given in two weeks; the health authority will seek advice from an independent panel which will consider the case. The panel will look at whether the health authority's eligibility criteria for NHS continuing care have been correctly applied, not question the criteria themselves.

Many NHS authorities have radically reduced the number of inpatient beds available for continuing care as more and more elderly people have been discharged to private nursing homes. The guidance suggests there may be a need for health authorities and general practitioner fund holders to reinvest in the provision of continuing care beds to meet the needs of patients who fall within the eligibility criteria. The beds may be provided within the hospital or contracted with the private or voluntary sector.

The new arrangements came into force in April 1996, and it is not yet clear whether more people will be judged eligible for NHS continuing care or if the appeal mechanism will work.

The future

If elderly people not eligible for public finance have to pay for their care in private nursing and residential homes, they may not be able to pass on wealth to their children. Thus the expectations of a generation of middle aged people that they would inherit sizeable amounts from the property values of their parents' home will not be met. This is a political issue, and time will tell if other funding for nursing home care becomes popular—for example, by private insurance schemes.

The future costs of long term care have been discussed in two recent documents—the House of Commons Health Committee report[34] and a report from the Joseph Rowntree Foundation.[35] The health committee emphasised the extreme difficulty of making reliable long term projections of costs; the Department of Health itself did not think that long term care was necessarily unaffordable, though pessimistic predictions forecast a fivefold rise in expenditure. There will possibly be considerable increases in costs, however, in the middle decade of the next century. Various options for financing long term care were discussed. At one end of the spectrum it was thought that the state should provide institutional and domiciliary long term care services free at the point of use. This would require considerable additional resources to be provided to local authorities by the government. The Royal College of Nursing has argued for the nursing element of long term care in nursing homes to be provided free by the NHS. Another possibility is to make all the costs of nursing homes the responsibility of the state. Another proposal is that all social and health care received in residential or nursing homes should be available free of charge, except for hotel charges which would continue to be means tested. The committee's preferred option was that the nursing costs of long term care should be met by the NHS, as this was the most equitable solution.

The committee also looked at incentives for people to make provision for some or all of their care. Two thirds of retired single person households have an income of less than £116 a week, with five out of six such households having an income of less than £61 a week. Therefore only 4% of those aged 75 and over would be able to meet residential fees from their income.

Release of money from capital assets is therefore the only way most older people can contribute to their own care. The committee did not consider that long term care insurance was acceptable, concluding that insurance policies of this kind are too expensive for most people. There is also a need for regulation of this market. Other options are partnership schemes to protect assets, although these are also too expensive for most people, and equity release schemes, to enable people rich in assets but poor in income to make provision for their long term care while protecting a proportion of their assets. The conclusion is that the status quo for funding long term care from taxation for those who cannot afford to pay should continue.

The Joseph Rowntree Foundation, however, found widespread criticism of the current system of funding long term care for elderly people when they surveyed a sample of the general public. People thought they had been given a false promise by the state that long term care for older people would be provided free at the point of delivery—the obligation to pay tax and National Insurance had led people to expect state funding of care. Means testing for residential and nursing homes was seen as unfair—thrifty people who had been careful and saved their money would have to pay for their care, while the spendthrift would be eligible for state funding. The idea of being forced to sell their home to pay for care caused great distress to people, who had hoped to leave it to their children.

It was widely thought that nursing care for older patients should be provided free within the service offered by the NHS. There were also objections to local authorities charging for domiciliary care services. People believed that revenue from supposedly dedicated contributions such as National Insurance had not been used for its intended purpose. Therefore any new system of tax or social insurance for long term care must carry an assurance that any revenue collected would be dedicated to a stated purpose, would be properly invested, and would guarantee the provision of a specified level of care. There was an acceptance of the need for some private insurance in the future, either for the younger generation in place of state funding or as well as state funding to pay for "top up" care.

A debate has therefore begun in society about how long term care for elderly people should be funded. This will certainly continue to be an issue for politicians in the future.

1 Royal College of Physicians of London. *Ensuring equity and quality of care for elderly people.* London: RCP, 1994.
2 Williams R. *Commissioning services for vulnerable people.* London: British Geriatrics Society/NHS Advisory Service, 1994.
3 Tallis R. Rehabilitation of the elderly in the 21st century. *J R Coll Physicians London* 1992;**26**:413–22.
4 World Health Organisation. *International classification of impairments, disabilities and handicaps. A manual of classification. Relating to the consequence of disease.* Geneva: WHO, 1980.
5 Young J. Caring for older people: rehabilitation and older people. *BMJ* 1996; **313**:677–81.

6 Mahoney FI, Barthel DW. Functional evaluation: the Barthel Index. *Maryland State Med J* 1965;14:61–5.

7 Royal College of Physicians. *Standardised assessment scales for elderly people.* London: Royal College of Physicians/British Geriatrics Society, 1992.

8 Wade DT, Callan FN, Robb GF, *et al.* Physiotherapy intervention late after stroke and mobility. *BMJ* 1992;304:609–13.

9 Sunderland A, Tinson DJ, Bradley EL, *et al.* Enhanced physical therapy improves recovery of arm function after stroke. *J Neurol Neurosurg Psychiatry* 1992;55: 530–5.

10 Smith DS, Goldenberg E, Ashburn A, *et al.* Remedial therapy after stroke: a randomised controlled trial. *BMJ* 1981;282:517–20.

11 Young JB, Forster A. The Bradford community stroke trial: results at six months. *BMJ* 1992;304:609–13.

12 Audit Commission. *United they stand—coordinating care for elderly people with hip fracture.* London: HMSO, 1995.

13 Neill J. *The discharge from hospital of people over retirement age.* London: Research Unit, National Institute of Social Work, 1987.

14 Victor CR, Vetter NJ. Preparing the elderly for discharge from hospital: a neglected aspect of patient care? *Age Ageing* 1988;7:155–63.

15 Williamson V. *Who really cares.* Brighton: Brighton Community Health Council, 1985.

16 Harding J, Modell M. Elderly people's experience of discharge from hospital. *J R Coll Gen Pract* 1989;39;17–20.

17 Williams EI, Finton F. Factors affecting early unplanned readmission of elderly hospital patients. *BMJ* 1988;297:784–7.

18 Department of Health. *Discharge of patients from hospital.* London: HMSO, 1989.

19 Department of Health. *Discharge of patients from hospital.* London: Department of Health, 1989. (HC(89)5, LAC(89)7.)

20 Henwood M, Wistow G. *Hospital discharge and community care. Early days.* London: Social Services Inspectorate, Department of Health, 1994.

21 NHS Executive. *Hospital discharge workbook, a manual on hospital discharge practice.* London: Department of Health, 1994.

22 Connor A, Tibbett JE. *Social workers and health care in hospitals: a report from a research study.* Edinburgh: Central Research Unit for Social Work Services Group, Scottish Office, 1988.

23 Iliffe S. Medication review for older people in general practice. *J Roy Soc Med* 1994;87(23):11–13.

24 Neill J, Williams J. *Leaving hospital, elderly people and their discharge to community care.* London: National Institute for Social Work Research Unit, HMSO, 1992.

25 Smith I, Easton P, Oliphant J. No significant change in discharges. *BMJ* 1994; 309:606.

26 Ajayi V, Miskelly F, Walton I. The NHS and Community Care Act 1990: is it a success for elderly people? *BMJ* 1995;310:435.

27 Lewis P, Dunn R, Vetter N. NHS and Community Care Act 1990 and discharges from hospital to private residential and nursing homes. *BMJ* 1994;309:28–9.

28 Social Services Inspectorate. *Moving on.* London: Department of Health, 1995.

29 Social Services Inspectorate. *Moving on: a further year.* London: Department of Health, 1995.

30 Millard P. Options in the NHS. *Health and Social Services Journal* 1988;94: 852–3.

31 Morris J. The case for the community geriatrician. *BMJ* 1994;309:127.

32 British Geriatrics Society. *Community geriatric medicine.* London: British Geriatrics Society, 1994.

33 NHS Executive. *NHS responsibilities for meeting continuing health care needs.* London: Department of Health, 1995. (HSG(95)8.)
34 Health Committee. *Long term care: future provision and funding, third report.* Vol 1. London: HMSO, 1996.
35 Joseph Rowntree Foundation. *Meeting the cost of continuing care: public views and perceptions.* London: Joseph Rowntree Foundation, 1996. (Social Care Research 84.)

7 What next?

In a climate of organisational instability and scarcity of resources the medical and social care of older people can be so problematic that clinical workers, managers, and providers of social care can become exhausted by trying to hold services together and maintain quality. Ideological "solutions" to problems—like "community care", the 75 and over checks, or care insurance for later life—become plausible in the absence of alternatives grounded in both experience and research. In this chapter we review the three areas of care for older people that we consider fundamental and offer some answers to the difficult questions posed. The three fundamental areas are: the development of skill in primary care beyond the 75 and over checks; the promotion of multidisciplinary and interagency working; and the future funding of medical and social care.

The development of primary care for older people

We have argued that the contractual obligation on general practitioners to offer annual domiciliary checks to all their patients aged 75 and over should be replaced by an approach to case finding and case management that exploits the potential of the information technology currently available (but underused). This approach could also be an obligation but a flexible one that is negotiated into the practice-based contracts that are likely to replace the standard individual contract and subject to audit and review. There

156

are two other developments, however, that could occur in primary care in parallel with this change—one preserving some element of active (if simple) health promotion for older people and the other closing the knowledge gap about disability.

A minimal health promotion package

Two very technical tasks undertaken by general practitioners and their teams can make an immediate difference to the health of older people: annual flu vaccination of older people and control of hypertension (see chapter 5). Both of these should be programmes that practices should implement as part of a package of health promotion activity and review critically in their annual reports. Annual flu vaccination is cheap, largely acceptable, and reduces the incidence of and mortality from major respiratory tract infections in older people.[1] Treatment of hypertension at all ages up to 80 reduces the incidence of and mortality from both heart disease and stroke, although general practitioners will need consciously to overcome a bias towards treating younger rather than older patients if these benefits are to be obtained.[2] Existing electronic medical records allow the uptake of flu immunisation and the extent and effectiveness of finding cases of hypertension and treating it in older people to be managed and audited relatively easily.

Five other common problems for older people could usefully be considered by primary care teams as themes for their work (see box on p. 158) but only in the context of evaluation of different approaches.[3] As research and development funds move towards primary care, general practitioners and their teams (together with staff working in community trusts) may have opportunities to mount such evaluation studies.

Attention to these problems within a framework of careful evaluation would help primary care workers to think about the needs and problems of their older population as well as their older patients, but translating sound evidence or even good intentions into lasting practice would require some deepening of understanding about disability and chronic disorders.

As a whole we health professionals are not sensitive to the personal and social consequences of chronic ill health and disability among our patients.[4] In particular, we:

157

- Are unaware of a substantial amount of disability
- Underestimate morbidity
- Misjudge our older patients' views on their quality of life.

Yet we also tend to visualise disability in later life as unrelenting decline, as do many of our patients.

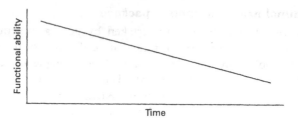

Fig 7.1

This conception of unrelenting decline can[4]:

- Dampen the expectations of professionals and patients alike
- Promote the emergence of such a pattern if behaviour is shaped by such expectations
- Shape service provision in such a way that dependence is encouraged to the detriment of patient and professional alike (for example, the development of residential care for older people with relatively minor functional loss)

Problem	Intervention
Osteoporosis	Dietary and vitamin D supplementation
	Screening with DEXA scanning
Iatrogenesis	Medication review
	Patient education
Depression	Case finding, counselling, and social engagement
Urinary incontinence	Case finding and intervention by continence nurse
Accidents	Home modifications

- Reduce efficiency through overprovision in the form of medication that is not taken and aids and appliances that are not used.

The actual course of chronic ill health can be very different, especially when considered from the viewpoints of the patient and his or her carers and may take a stepwise form or follow an unpredictable pattern.

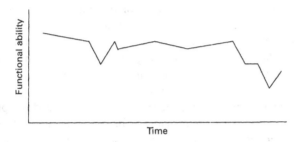

Fig 7.2

As we come to understand the variability of chronic ill health and disability a number of changes in practice can occur[4]:

- The need for flexibility and adaptiveness in services becomes obvious
- Some patients can become less dependent
- Demand for some services could decrease (as long as patients knew that services would be available if the need arose)
- "Crises" or downturns would not be surprising, and contingency planning could occur
- Feelings of self mastery can increase with an impact on the rate of decline itself
- Measures sensitive to improvement as well as decline become important.

Recent changes in the management of benign prostatic hypertrophy illustrate the difference that these two perceptions of chronic ill health can have on clinical practice. As all older men experience some symptoms of "prostatism" and have some degree of prostatic hyperplasia, the model of unrelenting decline predicts that all will need to undergo prostatectomy unless death from other causes supervenes. Demand for prostate surgery could therefore be modelled and service requirements planned. If, however, the course of benign prostatic hypertrophy is found to be unpredictable, variable judgments about the need for and timing of surgery become more complex, especially if new medical treatments for prostatic hyperplasia make improvements and remissions in the condition more common. In this scenario, the need for surgical intervention can decline, treatment options increase, and the emphasis shifts from solutions that "fix" the problem to knowledge that allows patient and doctor alike to make rational judgments. The scenario of demands this makes on the health service are very different from those made by the model of unrelenting decline because the former deals with familiar problems of logistics in a familiar production process and the latter with the interchange and evaluation of information by professional and patient.

Two needs emerge for professionals from these descriptions. One is the need to get the measure of health, illness, and disability among older people and the other is to have a shared understanding of the progress and process of chronic ill health and disability. While valid and reliable instruments currently being developed, like the Camberwell Assessment of Need (CAN), may be sensitive measures for the assessment of need among older people, they are unlikely to do more than augment enhanced professional judgment and skill. Understanding of the extent of the impact of disability and chronic ill health is fundamental, and promotion of this in undergraduate and postgraduate training in both general practice and nursing is a priority if professional practice is to change. Shared understanding of the impact of disability and of the progress of functional loss are linked and depend on the extent and depth of communication between professionals and patients—hence the emergent interest in the involvement of older people themselves in service change and development.

Reforms in primary care

General practitioners and other members of the primary health care team struggling with change all around them and increasing demands on their time are unlikely to see many opportunities for becoming involved in the evaluation of different approaches to common problems in later life, in focusing on disability and its impact, or on involving their older patients in reshaping provision and are likely to dismiss proposals for major changes in the ways in which they work. Before the changes announced in 1996–7 this attitude was justified, but the shift in resources towards the community and the dissolution of traditional organisational and professional boundaries promoted by the Primary Care Act *may* allow primary care workers to focus on the needs of their older patients and work together in ways previously difficult or impossible to achieve.

The primary care legislation of 1997 was preceded by three publications in 1996: *Primary care: the future,*[5] *Choice and opportunity,*[6] and *Delivering the future.*[7]

A primary care led NHS was restated as the cornerstone of policy. *Primary care: the future* was published for consideration by the NHS Executive after a listening exercise in the service. The principles of good primary care were identified in respect of quality, fairness, accessibility, responsiveness, and efficiency. General medical practice is recognised to be at the heart of the primary care system. The diversity of general practice is one of its strengths, along with the development of peer review, rigorous training and re-education, and flexibility in meeting patients' needs. There is, however, a need for greater consistency in the quality of care provided. Particular areas for attention are the provision of general medical services for severely mentally ill people, pressures on consulting time, the need for more primary care research, the use of contracting arrangements to promote and facilitate the processes of accreditation and reaccreditation, better information for patients, and greater emphasis on patients' responsibilities for their own health.

Primary health care should provide continuity of care; be comprehensive; be properly coordinated so that professionals work well together, if necessary in partnership with secondary care and other agencies, to meet a patient's needs; be the gatekeeper to secondary care, often through general practice; and deal with the health needs of communities as well as of individuals. Out of a discussion of a wide range of issues in primary care, covering all disciplines, a future agenda emerged.

There was a highlighted need for greater flexibility in the way funds are used—the division between general medical service and hospital and community health service funding was seen as increasingly artificial.

Partnerships in care need to be developed—there is a need for better team working between all the relevant primary care team members, with clear responsibilities for coordinating the care of individual patients, increasing the role of non-medical staff in providing care, and strengthening partnerships with secondary care, health authorities, and social services. Developing professional knowledge was seen to be important, with a greater proportion of basic and postgraduate training for all health care professionals (including vocational training of general practitioners) to be spent in a primary care setting. A greater proportion of all education and training should be multidisciplinary and continuing education should be developed. Patient and carer information and involvement should be increased, while recognising patients' responsibilities as well as rights.

The problem of recruitment to general practitioner training and general practice needs to be examined, with a different approach to contracts for general practitioners and promoting innovation in the way staff are used. The problem of poor and inflexible premises also needs to be dealt with. Linking practices together in various ways was seen to be a way of enhancing their individual and collective potential, and health authorities will have a key role in this development. There was a need for greater local flexibility and to allow innovative local ideas to flourish and be tested before they are more widely implemented. Many involved in the listening exercise thought that the time was right to bring about important changes to the contracts of general practitioners—for example, general medical services could be provided by a salaried service, with general practitioners employed by a community trust, a definition of core general medical services, and a split general practitioner contract between day and night services.

In October 1996 the Secretary of State for health published a white paper *Primary care: choice and opportunity*, setting out the government's intention to legislate on a number of key areas of primary care.[6] This enabled new approaches to contracting for general medical services—such participation should be voluntary, patients should continue to have the right to be registered with a general practitioner and to be able to choose their general practitioner, pilots should be evaluated, public accountability must be maintained, new arrangements are to emerge from the field rather than imposed from the centre, and there should be a facility to revert to the existing arrangements. Pilots can involve practice based contracts to include the primary care team, not just general practitioners; salaried general practitioners (in partnership with trusts); single unified budgets for hospital and community health services and general medical services; health authorities to negotiate with general practitioners; extended general medical services funded from hospital; and community health services—for example, management of chronic disease and mental health projects. Similar schemes are being invited for community pharmacy, involving them more in health promotion, providing advice for minor ailments, facilitating better use of prescribed medicines, and providing more advice on medicines to the rest of the primary health care team and to others. Similar changes are planned for dentists and optometrists.

Expressions of interest in new pilot projects to run a new type of service have been invited by health authorities. A timetable over the next year involving more detailed applications and local consultations has been set out and it is intended that pilots go live in April 1998. Full evaluations will be carried out after that time.

In December 1996 the government produced a second white paper on primary care—*Primary care: delivering the future*, setting out 70 practical proposals for action and details of some additional funding.[7] The existing nurse prescribing scheme is to be extended, and roles for health visitors, nurses, and midwives are to be developed. "Shared care" agreements between hospital ophthalmologists, general practitioners, and optometrists are to be piloted to enable general practitioners to direct patients with eye problems to optometrists and, when appropriate, for optometrists to refer patients direct to the hospital service (notifying general practitioners at the same time).

Team working is to be supported through specific training and information technology developments—for example, shared databases and electronic messaging—and contracts may now be placed based on practices not just general practitioners. This would allow a more flexible use of resources which would provide increased opportunities for multidisciplinary work and the use of skill mix between general practitioners, nurses, therapists, managers, and others.

Greater cohesion is needed, the white paper argues, between research, clinical audit, clinical guidelines, and professional education. Practice nurses are to be included in schemes for

163

improving professional education and training. A national salaried doctors scheme will be introduced for those who want it, and various changes to general practitioner training will occur. The legislation (NHS Primary Care Bill) received royal assent in March 1997 to enable the changes to take place.

So how may these changes affect services for older people? Three mechanisms could permit positive developments:

(1) Practices opting to provide secondary services could obtain resources to develop multidisciplinary teams for primary care of older people—initiated, but not necessarily led, by general practitioners with specialist input working alongside generalist services.

(2) Community trusts opting to provide primary care could introduce generalists into their existing specialist teams, allowing the development of primary care with a focus on older people within a broader organisation whose services spanned all ages and most needs.

(3) Acute trusts opting to provide primary care as an outreach facility associated with, say, their accident and emergency departments and outpatient clinics could create mixed specialist-generalist teams for the care of older people around existing "community geriatricians".

All three mechanisms could provide high quality care for older people, and each may be more appropriate in some settings than in others. Advanced *shire county* practices already experienced in fundholding may choose the first option, while in the inner cities the second and third options may be competitors.

Initiatives with community pharmacy could develop, enabling them to give more advice to individual patients and deal with patients' concordance with medicine regimens and to educate members of the primary health care team. Salaried general practitioners and dentists may be able to devote more time to elderly people; there are currently perverse incentives in the independent contractor status which militate against groups of more time-consuming clients. There is evidence that workload goes down (to more appropriate levels?) in salaried systems and this may encourage better multidisciplinary working. Support for multidisciplinary working through focused training, development of information technology practice-based contracts, and extended roles for health visitors and nurses may also improve care for older people.

There are some potential problems, however, and the pilots will need to be carefully evaluated. Diversity of practice could be good but may lead to inequity. Some pilots will be a form of market testing and could lead to fragmentation of the service, which always militates against good care for elderly people. The future of general practitioner fundholding is not clear with a change of government in May 1997, and locality commissioning will have to be strengthened to combat some of the levers for privatisation already in the system. There are no clear mechanisms for consumer or user involvement, and it is not clear how this market of care will be regulated. There is a problem of a disjunction between the policy and the operational view of practitioners, who are overloaded with perpetual change, rising workloads, and competing priorities, and may have individual concerns about their own place in the system and future career structure, for example.

Currently the hospital and community health service budgets are weighted (under the York formula) to try to direct resources to areas of highest morbidity. If the budget were to be merged with general medical service budgets this could mean money being moved out of some more well resourced practices to areas of greater need; while being more equitable this could obviously cause problems for existing practices and is likely to be strongly resisted by those practices who would lose out.

Another change which is taking place is a move to provide secondary care services in a primary care setting—individual general practices can apply to the health authority to provide such services in addition to the core general medical services. Bids will be judged by appropriateness and quality but services affecting elderly people particularly could include anticoagulation monitoring (for stroke prevention in patients with atrial fibrillation), endoscopy services, or possibly day hospitals.

The future of primary care is therefore difficult to predict, with many possibilities for change. It is important that services are developed to meet the needs of older people and to improve on the current provision; it remains to be seen if this will be the case.

Multidisciplinary and interagency working

The potential for redefining primary care itself may make previous hopes that general practitioners would learn "networking" as a mechanism for improving the care of older people[8] less important. While the idea of practices networking with other local agencies that contribute to services for older people is innovative, for professionals accustomed to "referral" as the main mechanism for obtaining care for patients it lacks depth when compared with the checklist for collaborative action shown below.[9]

The basic requirements for collaboration are:

(1) A negotiating process in which shared objectives can be developed as a basis for action

(2) Cycles of negotiation to deal with evolving objectives

(3) Objectives that motivate all participants, producing tasks that are enjoyable, challenging, and interesting

(4) High levels of participation, time to share information and ideas, and opportunities to influence outcomes

(5) A commitment to professional excellence, with mechanisms to manage constructive controversy

(6) Time given to innovative and constructive ideas

(7) Respect for different professional roles

This list may appear alien or unrealistic to many working in the NHS simply to maintain services for older people, but the requirements listed will need to become part of everyday working experience given the probable shape of health and social care for older people for the foreseeable future. We can assume that the pattern of care will include[4]:

● The involvement of several different professionals and non-professionals in the care of many patients, both inside and outside hospital

● The provision of care for individuals with chronic ill health from more than one organisation

● Management of acute illness episodes outside hospital

● More, but shorter stays in hospital for some care groups.

One response to this fragmentation of care within the NHS is to seek a "seamless service", but seamlessness may cause "bagginess"—excessive activity that is designed to foster collaboration but that, in fact, fails to meet individuals' needs. Tailoring of services may be a more appropriate analogy for those working with the sometimes complex problems of older people.[4]

How to tailor care? This may be obvious (if difficult given resource constraints) for individuals but what about groups—including older people in any given locality? The answer may lie in the kind of community orientation that is possible in primary care, using the kinds of approaches to needs assessment mentioned above in a cyclical process that identifies and prioritises problems, develops and implements responses to them, and evaluates their outcome.

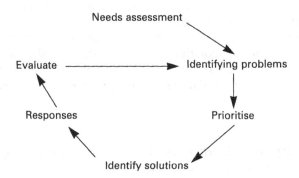

Fig 7.3

Application of the basic requirements for collaboration will need more than goodwill and the opportunities provided by the reform of primary care; training in multidisciplinary working needs to be developed.[10] Extra resources are needed to provide the time needed to allow in depth communication between patients and professionals and among professionals themselves; yet NHS expenditure for older people increased at a slower rate than for younger age groups between 1983 and 1993, the number of whole-time equivalent district nurses fell by 40%, as did all other types of community services for older people, although to a lesser extent.[11] The problem of funding needs to be solved if the developing awareness of how to collaborate in meeting the needs of older people is to be translated into effective teamwork and tailored care. Multiagency working at the level of health authorities, trusts, social service departments, fundholding general practitioner, locality commissioning general practitioners, and the voluntary sector is also essential. The managerial culture of collaboration must be fostered.

When funds are restricted there is a natural tendency for "cost shunting"—that is, to define circumstances where one agency will not meet the bill but expects the other to pick up the expenditure. An example of this is in definitions of eligibility for continuing care criteria—health authorities may wish to define certain categories of patients as *not* needing continuing health input, social services may define them as *not* needing social care but health care. Unless clear agreements have been reached, individual practitioners are involved in disputes on the ground, and there is a danger that individual clients are passed from one agency to another or slip through the provision altogether.

Communication at the highest level of agencies is needed and a commitment to collaborative working and the "seamless service". While these aims are laudable, many organisations have a long way to go before the ideal of true multiagency working is reached.

Funding health and social care for older people in the twenty-first century

Although only one in seven of the population is aged 65 or more, this age group accounted for 45.5% of Department of Social Services expenditure in 1993–4 and 40.5% of Department of Health expenditure.[7] This age group will increase by something like 34% in the next 35 to 40 years, and even though the great majority will not be in need of continuing medical or social care, the actual demand on services is likely to rise, and older people will find themselves competing with younger groups of the population even more than now for social and health care funding. The present arrangements for providing care are unjust because health services are essentially free at the time of need while social care and private nursing care require financial contributions (of various sizes) from their older recipients. In situations where an older person needs a place in a residential or nursing home or even intensive long term home care the prospect of wealth cascading down the generations recedes as the patient's assets are used up in providing the necessary care.

There are a number of possible responses to the funding of care for older people and although those of us involved in providing such care may not have any direct influence over funding policy, we can and should speak with the authority of experience about the difficulties created for individual older people and for agencies serving them by the present funding arrangements.

The continuation of the present divide between free health care and means tested social care would be unjust and divisive and in our view is not an acceptable option because it creates situations like that described in the case of Mrs M in chapter 6. The argument that wealth should cascade down the generations unaffected by the needs of the older person does not seem relevant to the debate as this view is highly contentious—why should it happen?—and would require considerable public subsidy of private affluence.

The costs of nursing care in nursing homes could be borne by public funds, leaving food and hotel costs in homes and social care in the community as means tested components of the service. (This view is favoured by the Royal College of Nursing.) Alternatively, accommodation and hotel costs could be charged for in all sectors, removing the anomaly of free care in NHS continuing care beds, with support for those on low incomes.

The debate about funding options now hinges on the balance between the social responsibility of aiding all citizens equally and individual responsibility for self care.[12] Two broad viewpoints exist in this debate. Long term care of any kind can be seen as akin to any other form of health care and should be provided free at the point of delivery. Payment of taxes and National Insurance should make any further payment by individuals unnecessary, and the whole population shares the costs of care for the minority of older people who need it. Alternatively, ongoing care in all its forms is different from acute care, scare resources should be targeted on those without the means to pay for themselves, and those individuals who have sufficient wealth should use it for their own long term care costs and allow the state to support the needy.

Each view begs a range of questions. Is there a limit to the amount of tax that can be raised? How much is the present generation prepared to pay to help previous generations? How much are we prepared to pay now to cover costs of our own possible care in the future? To what extent will the public in a consumerist society resist making any provision and instead stick with immediate gratification? Should people be compelled to make provision for their own future needs or is compulsion anathema in a free society? Should the private sector have an enhanced role in care provision or does the market produce more unfairness and inequity?

The demographic changes that are predicted for the next century may help us to work out the best policy option. Those over 85 have the highest need for continuing care and just under a quarter currently use nursing or residential home places. This age group will include 1.15 million in 2001 and probably about 2.2 million in 2041. Half a million will want or need institutional care in 2041, if present trends in disability and morbidity continue. Assuming that one third live at or below the poverty line (as now) and two thirds have some wealth in some form, about 170 000 people in this age group will need to contribute to their own care. If they are mostly living alone, their spouse having died, and on average had 1.5 children (being themselves children of the postwar baby boom who subsequently had small families), about a quarter of a million people would not inherit as much as they expected because of the care costs of the oldest old. These people may well have families with expectations of benefit, so that one or perhaps two million people would fail to gain their inheritance because residential care is means tested. Is their loss enough to justify making or encouraging a much larger group—all those now in their late 40s and upwards—set aside wealth for possible future care needs, perhaps through a compulsory National Care Insurance scheme as advocated by the Rowntree Trust.[8]

Perhaps those who fear the loss of inheritance should be responsible for insuring their parents? If they do so, they will in effect be paying an earmarked tax and transferring resources across the generations towards those most in need. This is exactly what happens now but through general taxation and returns us to the question of how much tax can be raised? The estimated cost of providing free social care in the home is currently about £100 million a year, while health and social care in nursing and residential home costs about £440 million a year, once adjustments are made for attendance allowance and means tested accommodation costs. Spread across 20 million employed people this amounts to an extra £27 a year in taxation. Not a bad premium to help keep the family silver and possibly even the family home in the family!

This compromise would mean that all accommodation charges for long term care would be levied from those who could afford them in both health and social care, while medical, nursing, and social care itself would be free. A commitment to home care would then be medically, socially, and economically sensible for all concerned, except for those who are hoping for growth in nursing and residential home care. Such a compromise would require extra funding for social, and to some extent for health services.

The teamwork needed to provide high quality home care would also needed pump priming, for it needs more staff time and more staff training than presently available if the working cultures of different professional groups are to change in the direction of collaboration and tailored care. The changes that might occur with a shift towards a primary care led NHS could help this, but the underdevelopment of knowledge and skills about the health of older people in general practice still needs to be put right, and no amount of reorganisation will do this. The resources to enhance general practitioner training (and arguably undergraduate teaching), to develop information technology that captures the complexity of health and illness in later life, and to install the audit mechanisms that will be essential to improving the quality of care need to be found. We hope that those who have read this book will be able to search them out successfully and make good use of them as we enter the next century.

1 Influences vaccinations and older people. *Effectiveness Matters* 1996; **2(1)**. York: NHS Centre for Reviews and Dissemination.
2 Ebrahim S, Davey Smith, *Health promotion for cardiovascular disease among older people*. London: Health Education Authority, 1996.
3 Ebrahim S. *'Tackling disease'—paper presented at the symposium 'Towards a framework for promoting the health of older people'*. London: Health Education Authority and Centre for Policy on Ageing, 1996.
4 Plamping D. *Developing better services for people with chronic illnesses—what are the issues?* London: Kings Fund, 1996
5 NHS Executive. *Primary care: the future*. London: NHS Executive 1996.
6 Department of Health. *Primary care: choice and opportunity*. London: HMSO, 1996.
7 Department of Health. *Primary care: delivering the future*. London: HMSO, 1996.
8 Edris Williams E, Wallace P. *Health checks for people aged 75 and over*. London: RCGP, 1993. (Occasional paper 59)

9 Standing Medical and Nursing and Midwifery Advisory Committees *In the patients interest: multi-professional working across organisational boundaries.* London: Department of Health, 1996.

10 Standing Committee on Postgraduate Medical and Dental Education. *Multiprofessional working and learning: sharing the educational challenge.* London: SCOPME, 1997.

11 Impallomeni M, Starr J. The UK Community Care Act (1990) and the elderly. *Lancet*1994;**344**:1230.

12 Joseph Rowntree Foundation Inquiry. *Meeting the costs of continuing care.* Rowntree Foundation, 1996.

Index

specialist services   17
  high quality   125–6
  mental health problems   124
  role of   142–6
staff, quality   126
supplementary benefits scheme   44–5

teamwork   88, 89, 130, 137–8, 163,
  171
telephones   66
training   29, 70, 162

transport, access to   7
treatment, responses to   10

urinary incontinence   104

values, underpinning care   31
vision assessments   103–4
voluntary organisations   13

Waltham Forest Hospital at
  Home   94